I, SPASTIC

The Autobiography of Neil Marcus

By Neil Marcus, with the able assistance of S. H. Chambers

BookStop Literary Agency LLC

Cover and Interior Design by Renata Galindo

Cover Photographs by Rod Lathim and Roger Marcus

1st edition 2024

Print edition ISBN: 979-8-218-47467-6
eBOOK ISBN: 979-8-218-47468-3

Library of Congress Control Number: 2024914933

Printed in the United States of America

Publisher's Cataloging-in-Publication data

Names: Marcus, Neil, author. | Chambers, S. H., author.
Title: I , spastic : the autobiography of Neil Marcus / Neil Marcus, with the able assistance of S. H. Chambers.
Description: Lafayette, CA: BookStop Literary Agency LLC, 2024.
Identifiers: LCCN: 2024914933 | ISBN: 979-8-218-47467-6 (paperback) | 979-8-218-47468-3 (ebook)
Subjects: LCSH Marcus, Neil. | Dramatists, American--20th century--Biography. | Authors--United States--Biography. | Artists--United States--Biography. | People with disabilities--Biography. | BISAC BIOGRAPHY & AUTOBIOGRAPHY / Entertainment & Performing Arts | BIOGRAPHY & AUTOBIOGRAPHY / People with Disabilities
Classification: LCC HV3013 .M37 2024 | DDC 362.4/3092--dc23

CONTENTS

A Note on Publishing This Posthumous Book

This book was many, many years in the making. When Neil set out to write his autobiography, he needed to sift through the boxed archives of his life, some dating back to the early 1980s.

To expedite the job, he teamed up with S. H. Chambers, a good friend from college. Neil chose the stories he wanted to add to his narrative and worked with S. H. to shape his experiences and thoughts into the manuscript. For three years, they traded drafts and messages online. But they hadn't quite finished when Neil died.

How to bring the book to a close? It is a challenging task when the author is not available to express opinions or answer questions. If he had had more time, Neil might have changed or cut passages. He might have chosen to end his story differently. But his time ran out.

Neil made it very clear that he did not want anyone to speak for him or alter his writing without his approval. S. H. had worked closely with him for so long that it made sense for him to complete the final chapter in Neil's absence. It is the only chapter that Neil had not seen.

Over the years, I, his sister, was Neil's 'go-to' person for everything from finding home healthcare providers to contacting doctors to discussions about marriage, love, and life.

The trust and mutual respect we developed over the years led him to assign the publication of this autobiography to me. I have shepherded the manuscript through the editorial process, through copyediting, and finally through design and publication. All along the way, S. H. served as my consultant, imagining how Neil would respond to the various decisions we faced as we sought to finish the book. I am confident that this is the story Neil wanted to share with readers.

—Kendra Marcus

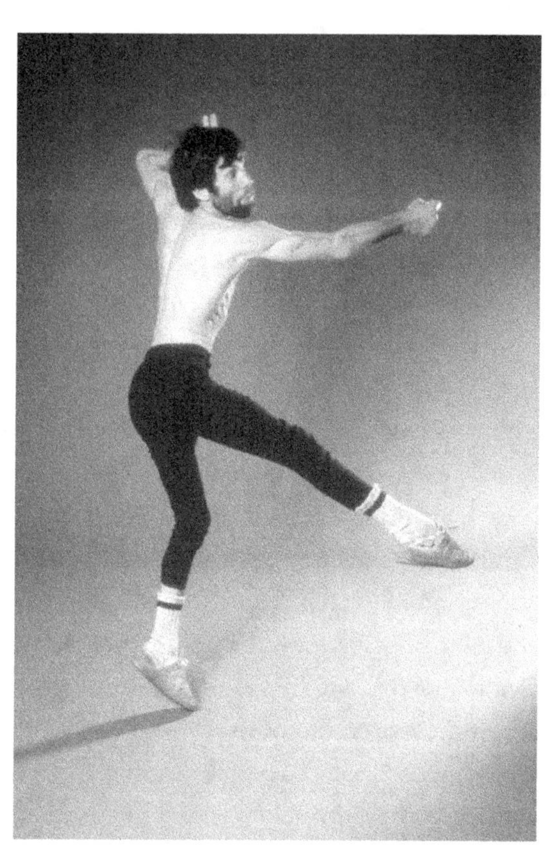

Disabled Country

If there was a country called disabled,

I would be from there.

I live disabled culture, eat disabled food, make disabled love,

cry disabled tears, climb disabled mountains,

and tell disabled stories.

If there was a country called disabled,

I would say she has immigrants that come to her

from as far back as time remembers.

If there was a country called disabled,

then I am one of its citizens.

I came there at age eight. I tried to leave.

Was encouraged by doctors to leave.

I tried to surgically remove myself from disabled country

but found myself, in the end,

staying and living there.

If there was a country called disabled,

I would always have to remind myself that I came from there.

I often want to forget.

I would have to remember…to remember.

In my life's journey,

I am making myself at home in my country.

—Neil Marcus (1980s)

I

From Here

Starting Point

1954

Disneyland will open next year.

❧

THIS IS SCARSDALE, A leafy village a few stops north of New York City.

And this is its hospital, where I was just born.

My birth is unremarkable. Ten tiny fingers, ten toes. My little heart is beating away. I take my first breath. Then I cry. There. All systems are good to go. I am a healthy baby boy.

I say my birth was unremarkable because healthy babies are born all the time. It's not that big of a deal. At the same time, it is amazing that babies are born at all.

Think about it. Each cell of the billions that are part of my pink little body must play its small part in performing the biological symphony that is my life. In a way, these cells have been in rehearsal for millions of years, evolving slowly through countless cycles of birth, love, and death. Still not amazed? Then consider this: who is conducting this orchestra of cells? Who is the composer of this living symphony?

Maybe no one is. I'm pretty sure it isn't me.

Here in the hospital, there is no sign of the cluster of cells that will do so much to shape the music of my life, no hint of what will one day be called my disability.

Here in Scarsdale, in 1954, I am a healthy baby boy, ready for the world.

Ready, willing, and able.

❧

We drive up to a big house with a wide lawn that runs all the way back to the woods.

I am home.

I meet my brothers and sisters: Roger, Wendy, Kendra, and Russell. Roger, the youngest, is already six. Wendy draws and paints. Kendra likes to read. Russell, the oldest, is almost an adult. He even sleeps in his underwear.

Every Sunday, the whole family listens to my mom's radio program. She makes up stories for children using three words chosen at random from postcards sent in by her listeners. She is called the Story Cook. One of my favorites is about a cow, a caveman, and a rocket ship. My dad spends a lot of his time resting. He had tuberculosis. And he makes movies for big companies.

I am the baby in a big, happy family. Everyone loves me, and I love them.

Soon, I am exploring: first on all fours, then, reenacting an important step in human evolution, I stand upright. Here I am, on two legs, wobbly at first, then steady. I stagger forward, swaying slightly. Suddenly, I am walking, and then running and running, around the house, past the swimming pool, across the lawn, through the apple trees, and all the way to the woods. Like there's nothing to it.

❧

I am four.

I am climbing on a jungle gym. I hang, I swing, I fly, and then, as gravity quietly asserts itself, I fall and break my arm.

So here I am, in a hospital bed, looking out on the corridor. My arm is in a cast. All the nurses are dressed in white. Even their shoes are bright white. One of them calls me "sweetie." The doctors all seem to be very suave and handsome, like superheroes. Hospitals are where mothers go to have babies and where kids have their tonsils taken out and then get to eat great mounds of ice cream. I am not that familiar with hospitals yet. The tedious medical subplot of my life story has not yet begun. Now, a hospital is a place where everything sparkles. Even the green Jello.

~

I am five.

My grandmother lives on a lake in southern Maine. Every time I visit her, she fixes me special sandwiches filled with sugar and a spread of butter. When I eat them on the porch, there is only the lake, the sky, warm bread, and sweetness.

There is a boathouse on the lake that fascinates me. Imagine a house that you drive into that has water as its floor. I love the sound of the water lapping against the sides as the structure shifts gently and creaks amidst the quiet of nature. And I love the smell inside the cool darkness of the boathouse. The lake water, the wet wood, and just a hint of gasoline, making rainbows in the water. It is just so wonderful.

The boat is made of shiny dark wood and has a silver horn mounted on the bow, in front of the windshield. This boat can pull water skiers, two at a time. Skiing on water is an incredible thing. That it works at all is just amazing to me.

~

Back home, I go over to a friend's house to watch TV. There's a trailer for a movie called *The Boy with Green Hair.* It's about this boy who wakes up one morning and all his hair has turned bright green. It is pretty scary. They've got a color TV.

In our backyard, in the evening, my attention is drawn to the fireflies and caterpillars making cocoons. Then my eyes follow the birds, and I notice the night sky.

I wake up in the dark. I get out of bed and walk down the hall to my parents' room. I go up to my mom's side of the bed and pat her arm. In the dim light, she blinks and asks me what's wrong.

"Mom, what's holding the stars up?"

A sense of wonder is drawing me outward, into a rapidly expanding world of beauty, mystery, and promise. In this world, hope has not yet become a device from which doctors dangle improbable cures, always just out of reach. In this world, hope is a warm feeling that good things are sure to come.

2

NEW FRONTIERLAND

Exploring Books and the Great Outdoors

1960

Next year, John F. Kennedy will become president.

WE ARE IN OJAI, A small town in a mountain valley about an hour north of Los Angeles.

We moved here because the clean, dry air will help my dad recover from tuberculosis. It rains less here, and the winters aren't nearly as cold as they are on the East Coast.

Our rambling redwood house is at the end of a long, curved gravel driveway on a big hill just outside of town. All around us are abandoned, decaying orchards and stands of oak and eucalyptus trees. It's an untamed place with snakes, hawks, and lizards. Our neighbor has a goat named Elsie.

I am six.

Most of the time, my brothers and sisters are away at boarding school or college. But I have lots of friends. I ride my bike down the hill into town to visit people I know.

To get to school, I follow an overgrown trail down the hill, across a dry creek bed, then past the ruins of a stone ranch house with fallen fences, broken wagons, and a derelict gas pump. The trail winds down to a road where I catch the van that takes me to school.

Jackie lives by the bus stop. She takes care of the horses in nearby pastures. I ask her if I can get a job helping brush the horses and she says okay. It's hard for me to do, holding the brush tight and keeping my balance when the horse moves. After a few days, I give up. I cry a little. I guess it was more than I could handle.

I am seven.

My best friend is Douglas. His family has a farm with a pond that has millions of tiny frogs swimming in it. They also have pigs that we feed oats and molasses. We try to ride a pig. It doesn't work.

After school and on weekends, Douglas and I play for hours, often staying outside until the darkness sneaks up on us. When the present is all there is, you lose track of time. It's like your clock stops ticking. When we do science experiments together at school, we wear white lab coats and call each other by our last names, Smith and Marcus. Very grown up.

Our science teacher takes us on a field trip to one of the dry riverbeds that tumble into Ojai Valley. Whenever it rains hard in the mountains, the water rushes down and turns barns into islands. The riverbed is filled with huge boulders and smooth stones that look like eggs laid by dinosaurs. I turn one over and find the underside still dark and damp from the last flood. Back at school, I make a slide of the gunk from under the stone and look at it through a microscope. We take turns looking at bacteria that haven't changed in a billion years.

I read a lot. *Swiss Family Robinson* and books by Jules Verne. I love the story of Samson. The Greek gods living on Olympus come alive as I read and reread about Zeus and Heracles and the rest. The way animals help humans in *The Jungle Book* amazes me. In my bed at night, I ride with King Arthur and the Knights of the Round Table on noble quests.

I watch movies, too. *Tarzan* is great, starring Johnny Weissmuller, and I watch anything with Boris Karloff. My brother Roger told me about this movie he saw called *The Fly*. It's about this guy whose DNA gets mixed up with a house fly's. At the end, there's a fly caught in this spider's web about to be eaten by the spider, but the fly has a man's head and arm. My mom says it really scared Roger. I couldn't believe it. Roger? Scared?

Our dog, Wy-mar, comes running whenever he hears me opening his daily can of dog food. Not other cans, just the dog food. I think he can tell by the combination of the sound and the time of day. I put his bowl on the floor, and he wolfs it all down in a flash. Two or three big gulps, and it's gone.

I often run from our house to our neighbor's. It goes like this: right at the beginning, there are fifteen boulders that serve as giant steps. I skip down from stone to stone. Every time, the same pattern, at the same speed. Dodge the cactus. Duck through the fence. Run across the big field really fast, before the horses notice. Under another fence, then comes a grove of tall eucalyptus to weave in and out of. And boom! I'm there.

I know what it means to have freedom in this body.

I know what it is to have a body that does what it's supposed to do, effortlessly. A body that rides bikes and leaps from stone to stone. I know what it is to have a body that is a seamless part of a family, a classroom full of kids, or a bunch of friends horsing around. A body that can move through a crowd of people with ease, even unnoticed, if need be. A body that fits.

I know what it is to be normal because I once was that which is still called normal.

3

A Bump in the Road

My Body Becomes Less Reliable

February 1962
John Glenn is in orbit, his body weightless.
A glitch pops up in the Mercury capsule.

❧

I AM EIGHT YEARS OLD.

During a pillow fight with Douglas, I sprain my right thumb. It's not a big deal. It hurts for a few days, then feels okay. But my hand doesn't move quite right.

"Give it some time," my mom says. "It'll get better."

A few weeks later, Douglas and I are caught swearing in class. I'm sitting outside the principal's office, and, what's this? My right wrist seems to want to pull my hand down. It's not really severe, but it's as though my wrist has begun to develop a mind of its own. Which seems pretty strange. The principal washes our mouths out with soap. It is an ordeal.

Writing becomes hard, then even harder, so I switch over to my left hand. This is a difficult thing to do. My mom does my science homework with me. We take turns writing, but even with practice, writing with my left hand doesn't seem to be getting any easier.

During recess, the most popular game is kickball. It's like baseball, but you kick a big rubber ball and then run around the bases. We play tag ball, too.

It's April now and not only is writing with my left hand not getting easier, but my left wrist also seems to be getting ideas of its own, too. It's tugging my left hand downward, bending it against my will. It's not too bad, not that strong of a tug, but still.

It's late spring, and I seem to have developed a slight tendency to limp. I mean, I can still walk, but what's going on here? Something is definitely going haywire. I try not to let anyone notice.

My parents take me to a doctor for some tests. He can't find anything wrong with my body that might be causing my limp or my bending wrists, so he talks to some other doctors, and they all agree that the problem is probably in my mind. They advise my parents to take me to a psychologist.

I'm in a big office with soft lighting and huge leather furniture. The wood paneled walls are lined with shelves full of thick books and decorated with framed diplomas and ornate plaques.

The psychologist is smoking a pipe that he tends to with this little tool that has these metal bits that scrape, clean, and tamp. From the way he looks at me, I can tell he's thinking really hard about what's going on with me, trying to figure it out. His eyebrows keep wiggling.

As we play some games with wooden blocks and pegs, he asks me, "How's life been treating you? Is there anything you'd like to talk about?"

He sounds really friendly.

Now he is trying to hypnotize me by swinging his gold pocket watch in front of my eyes, but I'm not a very good subject. Instead of getting hypnotized, I keep thinking that this is part of a script. It feels very strange to me, like I'm in a movie.

He takes me into a dimly lit room, and he asks me about using "forbidden" words. Then he asks me to say a bunch of swear words, over and over. Okay, but some of them are the same ones that got Douglas and me in trouble.

This whole experience doesn't feel quite real.

The psychologist tells my parents that they have been too nice to me. He says that they should quit treating me like a baby and toughen me up. He says that could help me to snap out of it. Or, he says, it might have something to do with sex.

What is he talking about? I just want my body back.

Then he suggests that my parents enroll me in a private school down the valley. It's pretty late in the school year, but he thinks the change might be good for me.

My dad and I go to the private school to meet Mr. Burr, the headmaster. He is tall, his hair is white, and his necktie is black. The way he stands makes me think of pictures I've seen of Abraham Lincoln. He and my dad talk over whether the school would be right for me. Mr. Burr sounds annoyed. Not at me. He sounds like he's annoyed at everything. He asks me a few questions. Finally, he comes to a decision.

"Yes. I think our school would be a good fit for Neil."

The all-powerful Zeus has spoken.

Back in the car, I wonder what Mr. Burr meant by "a good fit." I want to believe him, to have hope. But I can't. I tremble and cry, constricted by my fears.

4
From Behind The Bushes

Limping

May 1962

The Miracle Worker just came out. Patty Duke plays Helen Keller.
The Isley Brothers sing "Twist and Shout."

~

At my new school, it feels like I'm on a secret mission to hide my limp from my new classmates. I'm pretty sure that I have a cloak of invisibility that helps me to move among them unnoticed.

Every morning, all the boys and girls march single-file into the auditorium, singing together. One of the teachers accompanies us on a piano. It is always the same song. I sit as close to the door as I can to help ensure my invisibility. If I were to move farther into the room, I would risk being seen.

Land of Hope and Glory, Mother of the Free,
How shall we extol thee, who are born of thee?
Wider still and wider shall thy bounds be set;
God, who made thee mighty, make thee mightier yet.

The music of this song sounds solemn. And the words make it sound like it's about something really important. But what does "extol" mean? And "thy bounds be set?" What does that mean? I don't know. And this song doesn't seem to have very much to do with me keeping my foot straight, does it? Or me keeping people from seeing me? I mean, I'll sing the song, but to me, it's more or less just a bunch of words strung together.

I put on my cloak and leave the auditorium while everyone's eyes are still turned to the front.

The school is four buildings built around a large square courtyard. Whenever it's time to change classes, I wait till everyone else is in class, then hurry across the courtyard, careful to stay behind the bushes and trees. Hiding myself is a full-time job.

I do the same thing at lunch. I let everyone go ahead, so they can't see me walking. It means I have to sit wherever there's still a space in the lunchroom. Like musical chairs.

Sometimes I have to wait on tables. There's a chart on the wall that says whose turn it is to be the waiter. I don't like doing it. When it's my turn, I have to go up and down the rows, serving food to the other kids, walking as evenly as I can. Handing out rolls, or apples. The cooks, older women in aprons and white hats, watch me from the kitchen, their arms folded in front of them. It is a test of my bravery. I pretend not to notice them.

At the lunch table, I talk with my classmates. We joke around. But when I eat, my hands, my mouth, and my tongue don't move quite the way I want them to. It's like they're getting ideas of their own, too, and all I can think about is whether the other kids are watching me. I feel like I'm the star of a show that I don't want to be in. Hiding is my new reality.

And, well, it seems to be working.

So far, no one has said anything to me about how I walk. No one has mentioned how I eat either. No one seems to have noticed. Not the teachers, not the students. It seems strange, though, because I sure notice it. Then it occurs to me that maybe they're just trying to be nice to me. By not mentioning it.

I do not find this thought comforting.

Last night, there was a movie in the school's auditorium. In the movie, this guy is exposed to a mysterious cloud. Before long, he notices that his clothes seem to be getting looser, and at first, he thinks he's just losing a little weight. But then he gets smaller. Before you know it, he's three feet tall. There's absolutely nothing he can do. He becomes an overnight media sensation and a member of a circus troupe. He gets even smaller. Pretty soon, he moves into a dollhouse. The family cat attacks him. His wife leaves him. Smaller still, and he is hunted by a giant spider. It's called *The Incredible Shrinking Man.*

At the end, when he's so tiny that no one can see or hear him, the camera zooms in for a close-up. He turns and looks right at me and says something like, "The world wants you to believe that you are insignificant. But you're not, no matter what," and then steps into the subatomic mist.

I did not enjoy this movie.

The psychologist tells my parents and me that the thing that's causing my wrist and my toe to turn is my subconscious. I don't know what that is. My mom and my dad don't tell me. I guess they think I already know. I ask Roger. He is 14. He probably knows what a subconscious is.

"It's sort of like there's this part of your brain that's naughty," he says. "And it tries to make you do bad things. It's like it's talking to you, and you can't really hear it, but you sort of can? I saw it on *The Twilight Zone.*"

This isn't good.

The psychologist says that my parents and I should schedule regular sessions with a psychotherapist to get at the root of the problem in my subconscious.

So here I am, in another wood-paneled office with more huge leather furniture. This therapist doesn't have a pipe. He is a very kind man with a big beard and a soft, low voice who talks with me for a long time. Then he tells my parents that they should send me to summer camp. They both look at him, then at me.

"It might help," he says, "It might give him a whole new lease on life."

5
METAMORPHOSIS

What I Did Last Summer

Summer 1962

Andy Warhol's *Campbell's Soup Cans* are being shown in Los Angeles.

～

I'M STILL EIGHT, AND I'm going to camp for three weeks.

I'm at the Santa Barbara station, waiting for the train. My parents are here to see me off.

My dad puts a penny on the track. A train roars by. He picks the penny up and puts it in my hand. It's still warm. It's no longer a circle, perfect in its symmetry. It has been transformed into something like a giant squashed kidney bean. Abraham Lincoln's head is all stretched out, distorted. It isn't really a penny anymore. I mean, it won't fit in a gum machine. Instead of being a coin, the train has turned it into an ornament, an oddity, or maybe a talisman. My dad says it's my good luck piece.

"Hold onto it."

～

A rattly old bus takes me from the Redding train station to Silver Pines Camp, on the shore of a mountain lake surrounded by a forest. I step down from the bus.

Sure, I have a slight limp and, yes, my handwriting isn't that great. But I can do all the things you need to do at camp. I can walk and run, sort of. I'm a good swimmer. And I can sail and maybe even ride a horse.

I look around. A bunch of guys are swimming. A sailboat is cutting through the sparkles on the lake and behind it, peeking over the hills, is Mt. Shasta, still sporting snow.

The doctors say that the problem is in my mind. Well, what better place is there to toughen up and snap out of it than right here? I have three weeks.

I'm going to do this.

∽

I am sailing my dinghy. Out here alone, I have a sense of total freedom. I can go anywhere. I sail all over the lake, like Odysseus. Or like Magellan, sailing around the world.

I swim out to a raft in the middle of the lake to earn my certificate. While I'm swimming back, somehow I veer off to the left. Maybe I was blown off course by the wind. I'm not worried though, I'm tough. I end up way to the south of the camp and have to walk back along the shore through the tall trees, shivering, barefoot on pine needles. No one noticed I was gone.

Tonight, at the campfire, a counselor told us a story. This kid is kidnapped for ransom, but his parents refuse to pay. The kidnappers put the kid's head in a vise and each day that the ransom isn't paid they make it a little tighter. His parents still won't pay. They follow the advice of the cops and never pay. Now the kid is a young man and lives in the forest. He has a squashed head and comes out at night to fight against crime and injustice. His friends, the insects, help him. Big swirling clouds of insects of every color.

After the campfire, back in the dorm, guys take turns telling scary stories in the dark. It's my turn and in my most serious voice, I tell them that there are things I shouldn't talk about, mysterious forces that are at work, invisible connections between the mind, the body, and the unknown. Secret, forbidden things. Horrible things that do not even have names in this world. They think I'm making it up.

I'm having a little trouble getting to sleep tonight.

In the woods at Silver Pines, there is a kind of snake called a rubber boa that looks like a giant earthworm. I really wanted one and this morning, on the last day of camp, one came right over to me, as though I'd called it. The whole thing seemed like a story right out of *The Jungle Book*. The snake was gray and almost a foot long. I picked it up and put it in my pocket. It found a hole and slithered into the lining of my coat. I wondered if I have a supernatural ability to communicate with animals, like Tarzan.

As the train pulls into the Santa Barbara station, I see my parents on the platform, smiling at me and waving. I wave back. As I get down from the train, their smiles freeze, then morph into looks of concern.

I am hopping down the steps on my left leg, grabbing the handrail with both hands and dragging my right leg behind me. In an effort to avoid any more unpleasant surprises I say, "Ah. Habba. Rubba. Boan. Mah. Jakka." Their looks of concern turn into looks of shock.

I repeat the message, more slowly, adding gestures. They are not in the least bit reassured, in part because I'm having muscle spasms all over my body, jerking my limbs and twisting my torso, and in part because they have no idea what I'm trying to say.

I try a variation. "Ah. Habba. Snay. Kan. Mah. Jakka."

A light bulb switches on. My father says, "You have a snake in your jacket?"

"Yeah."

While I am pleased that he has understood me, he doesn't seem to be.

Both he and my mom are now looking at me with something approaching horror. A loving horror, of course, but horror, nonetheless. I can tell from their faces they now believe that, in addition to having lost control of my voluntary muscles and the power of speech, I have lost my mind. It is clear to me that my parents, at this moment, think that their baby boy has flipped out.

Using all my remaining credibility and powers of persuasion, I convince them to initiate a snake hunt. A few moments later, my dad pulls the rubber boa out of my jacket, just like in a magic show.

My parents are, of course, relieved. Their horror fades back into mere shock.

~

Why were they so surprised? Well, when I boarded that same train three weeks before, I had climbed the stairs with an air of confidence and a slight limp. Now, I can barely walk.

At camp, I could tell that I was losing my ability to control my movements, but I didn't really understand it. I was pretty sure that I should keep it a secret, that I should hide it from everyone, both kids and adults. Like walking behind the bushes.

I had become pretty good at hiding such things. If you're having trouble eating, eat things that don't need a lot of chewing, and eat as little as possible. Fill your pockets with things to eat later when alone. If you're having trouble talking, use gestures or give one-word answers. If you're having trouble walking, sit. When you're sailing a boat, no one can tell if you have a limp. If you're sailing alone, there's no one to hear you talk. And swimmers don't limp. Or talk.

People tend to look away from things they don't want to see. Everyone does it. The people at camp probably did. Besides, they didn't really know me well enough to figure out how big the change was. In their weekly reports to my folks, all they said was, "Neil is doing fine."

People want everything to be right, and if it's not, to make it right, but there are some things that are just beyond our control. There are times when we just have to accept reality.

I am standing with my mom and dad on the platform of the Santa Barbara station. My dad hands me the rubber boa. I carefully put it back in my coat pocket. The reality that my parents and I are now coming to grips with is that nobody is going to just snap out of anything.

6

FITTING IN

In the Mainstream

Spring 1963

The Beatles release their first album, *Please, Please Me*.

~

I AM NINE YEARS OLD. I'm on my bed in Ojai. My body is twisted, like the branches of the mulberry tree outside my window. I've been back at the same school since September. I'm in fourth grade. Things are different now. I can't walk or talk very well at all, or even button my pants.

On the first day of school, my dad came into the classroom with me. He was wearing a dark suit. And a necktie. He never wears a suit—not since we moved to California, anyway. He stood in front of the class to talk to the kids. Parents don't do this. Talk to the class. They just don't.

"Neil is fine. His arm or his leg may suddenly shoot out, but that's just because he can't control his muscles properly. And he's having trouble talking clearly. He's not doing it on purpose, and you shouldn't treat him any differently than you did last year. He's still Neil. Just treat him the same as everybody else."

22

My face turns red with shame. What he's saying isn't true. I am not the same kid I was. I don't really understand it, but I know it's real. I am different.

What are the other kids thinking? What are the teachers thinking? Are they thinking, "Oh, it's so sad. Poor Neil." I can't stand it. My dad is trying to help, trying to fix the problem, but how does this help? How could his little speech possibly fix anything?

PE class always starts out with everyone running a lap around the track, to warm up. On the first day, I tried, but I was having problems with my legs. I finally figured out that if I went backwards, I could make some headway. It wasn't easy, and it wasn't running, but it worked.

The next day, I was all set to do it again when the coach came over. With a casualness that was not yet familiar to me, he said, "No, not you. You don't have to." It seemed that he had been talking to my folks.

Not long after, my dad borrows a big, clunky wheelchair from the Easter Seal Society. It doesn't fit me. I don't want to use it. But they make me use it. Wheelchairs can't even go up steps, or down. I don't like this wheelchair at all. To me, it is my monster. Whenever I sit in this wheelchair, I can feel it wrap around me and then, suddenly, I'm fully visible, in all my shame and fear. It makes me ugly. I don't want my brothers and sisters to see me like this. I really hate it.

I am now what is referred to as a "handicapped child in a mainstream setting." In fact, I am the only "handicapped child" in the whole school. I am expected to "fit in." It is manageable, I guess. I have my daily routines. It doesn't seem like anybody is making that big deal of it. But "fitting in" isn't so easy, and I'm still trying to hide.

Older kids help me with the stairs now. They're past the point of pretending not to notice me and I've reached the point where I can accept help from them, even though it still hurts when I do. I have a different body now, a new body. Having a new body can change your outlook. A lot.

Even the bullies don't pick on me anymore. The other day, one of them, one of the really mean ones, came up to me and was actually nice. He even offered me some of his Fritos. It made me cry.

I'm not eating enough now. It's hard to chew and harder to swallow. I don't eat in the cafeteria anymore. Every day, either my mom or my dad comes to meet me at school during the lunch break and at recess to give me snacks to eat in the car. Then they help me use the bathroom and wheel me to the next class. The bathroom stalls are too small for the wheelchair and there's nothing to grab on to. My parents are allowed to help me take tests and write reports, too.

When we sit in the car, we listen to the radio. Sometimes, the emergency alert system is tested. It makes a long, high-pitched sound. *Eeeee.* They'll use it to warn people if the Russians attack America with atomic bombs. When it's over, a guy always says, "This was only a test." Once, I asked my mom what he would say if it wasn't just a test.

"What. If. It. Was. Real? What. Would. He. Say. Then?" I asked her. I really wanted to know.

She was behind the wheel, holding a spoon in one hand and a cup of applesauce in the other. At first, she didn't say anything, just looked at me with her brow slightly knitted and the hint of a smile. Then she said, "I don't know. But whatever he said, it would make all our other troubles suddenly seem very small."

My invisibility cloak isn't working very well, and I have become very shy. Taking the annual school picture is a nightmare. Everyone else is standing together in a line. I'm off to one end, sitting in the chair. It's the only place I fit. All the feelings of being strange rise up in me. It's like a form of torture.

Instead of hiding my limp, now I'm trying desperately to hide myself, wheelchair and all. Smile!

My view of this small town is different now, too. I don't like to ride into town with my mom anymore. Driving down the street by our house is now like running a gauntlet. People in their yards or walking on the street or kids playing now seem threatening to me. I always wonder if they're feeling sorry for me when they're out washing their cars, smiling, and waving cheerfully.

"Hiiiiii!"

A woman named Gladys lived at the bottom of the hill, at the corner. When she is out gardening or walking her dog and we drive by, she waves and greets me. Then one day I hear she'd been taken away because she thought the electricity in her house was attacking her. I feel sad for her. I think she was lonely. I think she felt as though she had a special connection with me.

"Hi, Neil! Hi!"

I only have one friend now, Leif. He lives just down the hill and is the same age as me. When I play with him, the edge of my shame feels dull. His family follows the teachings of Krishnamurti.

Mostly, I just stay at home. I feel safer on my hilltop. After I read *Silent Spring*, I get really upset about all the pesticides being used in the world. It reminds me of the mysterious cloud that made the incredible shrinking man shrink. It makes me feel that nowhere is safe anymore, that the whole world is a dangerous place. That there's nowhere to hide.

I do go to the park a lot. Either my mom or my dad takes me.

We play miniature golf. My technique is unconventional, but effective.

I also shoot arrows with a bow, like Odysseus shooting through the holes of the ax heads. My mom always looks a little nervous when I draw the bow, but I'm pretty good. Like Robin Hood.

And I go skateboarding. Yes, I just sit on the board, not stand. And, yes, for some reason it is easier facing backward, not forward. It's something about the center of gravity. I haven't rammed into anything yet.

Sometimes my dad and I fly kites over the valley. We tie the kites to our fishing poles. It works great. Sometimes we write a note and attach it to the kite line and send it way up into the sky. Like a wish. We love flying kites. Soaring, weightless.

Last week, we went to Disneyland. Roger and I rode in a boat together on the ride "it's a small world." We got to go to the front of the line because I was in a wheelchair. At the start, the attendant told us to keep our hands out of the water, but Roger put his hands in anyway. When we got out of the boat, he shook the attendant's hand. The attendant gave Roger a look that seemed out of place in the happiest place on earth.

I told Roger about my fears. He told me how much the movie *The Fly* had scared him. Especially the scene where the housefly with the man's head and arm calls out, "Help me! Help me!" He said I shouldn't be afraid.

The thing is, when I'm afraid, the spasms are worse. Doesn't that sound like a mental problem? Like it's in my mind? Well, if it is, I must be totally crazy, because a lot of the time my whole body is tied up so tight, I can't even pick up a pencil.

∼

My mom comes into my room and sits on the edge of the bed. I am on my side, my whole body clenched, arms and legs curled up, my head pressed against my chest. She places her hand on my shoulder. I am looking at her out of the corner of my eye.

I dare to ask the question. I dare to speak the words. I know that it is beyond what anyone can answer. I ask anyway, with great difficulty, forming the words very slowly.

"When. Will. I. Be. Better?"

For what seems like a long time, she doesn't say anything. Then she answers, very calmly, her voice sounding soothing and confident.

"Someday they'll come up with answers for you."

She doesn't cry, but I see tears in her eyes. I feel my own tears cross the bridge of my nose on their way to the pillow.

I'll never bring it up again.

7
"RIDE SHARING"

My Problem Has a Name

Summer 1963
Martin Luther King delivers his "I Have a Dream" speech.
President Kennedy will go to Dallas in the fall.

~

I'M STILL NINE.

Now, I mostly see the world from the back seat of a car. What interests me most are the fields beyond the fences. I look at them and think that if I could just get over that fence and if I just had the means, I could go wherever I want. I could be free.

~

I'm in downtown Santa Barbara, riding in the back seat. My folks are in front. We stop at a traffic light. Right outside my window are a bunch of hitchhikers with their thumbs out. One of them has curly red hair and is holding a sign. "San Francisco." He can see me through the window, sitting somewhat twisted up on the back seat.

I feel guilt. We aren't going to be giving him the ride he needs. He keeps looking at me. I look back at him out of the corner of my eye, my head down on my chest. And, I don't know why, but I feel intimidated. No, scared. Scared that he wants to judge me. And I ask myself again: am I crazy? Is being scared of hitchhikers part of the same problem that is twisting my body?

Then I feel fear rising in me. It is the fear that you feel in a horror movie. Only this isn't a movie. The fear makes the spasms stronger, which in turn feeds the fear, turning it into the kind of fear that grips your throat, the kind that you can taste. This is real.

Part of my mind is beyond my control, no matter what I do. No one knows why. I look up at my parents, looking out the front window. They want to help me, but they can't. No one can help me. I am alone. I have to fight this battle inside my head alone. I look at the red light and feel a chill pass through me as beads of sweat form on my forehead. And then I think of Dr. Frankenstein's monster, chased by angry villagers carrying torches and pitchforks.

The light changes.

～

It's still summer. I'm with my folks in the office of Dr. Rosner, in Los Angeles. He's behind a giant mahogany desk. It's like it's his castle and he's the king, and I'm a serf who needs his help. Then I notice that he has a heavy steel brace on his right leg. He is lame, like Hephaestus, the Greek god who is a blacksmith. Or like Festus, in *Gunsmoke*.

Dr. Rosner and I play some games. "Snap your fingers. Okay. Stick out your tongue. Wiggle it as fast as you can from side to side." He demonstrates. He can wiggle his tongue like a real pro. I can't. Mine is thick and slow, uncooperative.

After all the games, Dr. Rosner sits in his leather chair behind his giant desk and asks us to be seated across from him. He tells us what has been happening to me for more than a year now. He says I have a rare neuromuscular condition called *dystonia musculorum deformans progressiva*. He sounds like a wizard trying to cast a spell.

It is physical, he explains, not psychological. It is my body, not my mind, that caused my wrist to twist and my toe to turn inward. It is my body that is tying me up so tightly. I may be only nine, but even I know that, in a way, this is good news, both to me and to my parents, who had been accused of babying me, who had been told that it might be their fault.

He tells us that in the relay switches in my brain that route the messages being sent to my muscles, telling them when to contract and when to relax, some of the wires are crossed. It is these crossed wires, this neurological quirk, not some childhood fear or mysterious dark force, that makes my muscles spasm. The messages being sent are just getting scrambled by these rogue nerve cells, making opposing muscles contract at the same time.

He doesn't say so, but it also means I'm not crazy. My folks and I feel a sense of relief.

Then he tells us the bad news.

He tells us that dystonia doesn't just go away by itself. It sticks around. And over time, he says, its effects are not good. Not good at all. Dystonia takes a real toll on the body, especially in the joints, where the bones meet.

While we are still wrapping our minds around this news, Dr. Rosner tells us that there is a surgical procedure that sometimes helps reduce the number and strength of the spasms.

Sometimes it even stops them altogether.

It works like this: They drill a hole about the size of a dime in your skull and stick a long needle into your brain. Then they make the tip of the needle really cold and see if the right muscles relax. When they find the right place, they make the tip of the needle a lot colder to freeze the brain cells in that spot. If everything goes just right, when it's over, the muscle spasms are gone.

He tells us that this surgery is called a cryothalamotomy. More Latin. Abracadabra.

But the procedure is very difficult and unpredictable. It doesn't always work. Sometimes it doesn't help at all. And sometimes, not very often, he says, but sometimes, it can actually make things worse. Much worse.

⁓

My folks and I are back at home now, sitting at the big round table in our family room. We are facing a difficult decision.

I can't walk. It is really hard for me to talk. Using the bathroom is a big problem. It is hard for me to eat enough food. Hard to chew it. Hard to swallow. I'm getting really skinny. I spend a lot of time curled up in a tightly flexed ball.

I am ashamed of being different, of being seen as some kind of medical object. The worst thing, though, is to be pitied. I really hate it. If surgery could just put a stop to that, it would be worth it.

My folks tell me that when I wasn't there, Dr. Rosner said that without the surgery I could end up in a care facility and that I might not even live to be twenty years old.

But the surgery is very risky. It might make things worse. I might not even live through it.

In the end, we decide to take the risk. I'm going to have brain surgery.

8

DUNGEON

Pre-op Prep

Late 1963

American soldiers are being sent to Vietnam.

Roy Orbison sings "In Dreams."

⁓

BEFORE THE SURGEON picks up his scalpel, I have to try every medicine that has any chance at all of helping me.

Every day, my parents set up a row of shot glasses. In those glasses are my pills for that day. When it's clear that one medication isn't helping, another is prescribed. This goes on for months.

Most of the names of the medications are in Latin: benztropine, methyldopa, carisoprodol, diphenhydramine, scopolamine. There are lots more. They sound like alien life forms.

"It's a Scopolomine battle cruiser, Commander!"

Some of the pills make me sleepy, even a little woozy. A few of them just make me barf.

Anyway, it turns out that none of them work. But they're not through with me yet. There are other tests. Blood tests. Heart tests. And psychological tests. I actually like taking most of these tests. For me, they are outings. I don't have to go to school.

There was one test, though, that was definitely not a picnic.

My dad waited in my hospital room as the orderly wheeled me down the hall and into the elevator. When the doors opened, we were in the basement. We headed down the hall to an open doorway.

As we entered, two men wearing long white coats were bent over some equipment on a cart. One of them looked up at me, then back at the cart. His eyes were steel-gray, his hair was black and long and uncombed. The room was small, chilly, and windowless. A faint smell of harsh chemicals hung in the air. In the center of the room was a large wooden table with a thin blue foam pad on top.

After the orderly left, the long-haired guy said, "Larry, help this young man up."

Larry came over. When he grabbed my arm, then my ankle, his grip was really tight. "Up you go," he said, in a voice too loud for the tiny room.

As he strapped down my knee at an uncomfortable angle, I saw that his hands were thin and pale. His eyes never met mine. He held me while the long-haired guy came over and said, "This might hurt," and stuck a big needle into my right hip.

It hurt like stepping on a nail. I silently yelled, "No! Stop!" as he stuck another needle into me, this time, into my right calf. Still silent, I screamed, "Monsters! I'm right here! Can't you see what you're doing?!"

The needles in my leg were attached to wires that led back to a gray metal box on the cart. A black cord snaked from the box toward the wall. My eyes opened very wide.

It was plugged in.

Larry kept on holding me while the other guy fiddled with the box.

Then the long-haired guy looked over at my leg, looked back at the box, and threw a switch that gave me an electric shock.

The first one didn't hurt much, but he kept on turning up the knob and throwing the switch until each shock was really hurting me. I did not scream. I decided to just take it, but the voice in my head was screaming, "I'll have my revenge! You just wait!" As the shocks continued, and the strap cut into my leg, I silently called out, "Dad! Dad! Mom! Mom! Stop them! Someone, help me! Help!" Screaming out loud was not an option. The two men were busy looking at the dials and meters, and at my leg, and didn't notice that I was in pain.

Then he threw the switch again and my whole body gave a powerful jerk. Larry held on tightly, and the long-haired guy turned quickly and fixed his steel-gray eyes on me. I glared back.

They stopped the test. Maybe it was that spasm. Maybe that's how they know when the test is over.

When the orderly wheeled me back to my hospital room, there was my dad, sitting on the bed, doing the New York Times crossword puzzle. He looked at me, then said, "Neil, what's wrong?" I didn't say anything. I held it in. But as soon as the orderly left, I broke down, sobbing, my chest shuddering, my shoulders shaking. My father held me as I wailed out my pain, my fear, my helplessness, my shame.

I wailed in rage. "What. Are. They. Trying. To. Do. To. Me? It. Hurts! They. Are. So. Mean!"

My dad tried to comfort me. "They have to be sure the problem is with your body before they can do surgery." He was trying to keep his voice calm, but I could hear his anguish.

Through my tears, I said, "Not. Good. No. Reason. To. Jab. Me. They. Hurt. Me." Between my sobs and spasms, it took a long time to get this out. I wanted him to know.

We drove home. I was crying, curled up on the back seat. By the time we got to Ojai, I was mostly cried out.

On a day trip to LA, my parents and I took a tram tour of the back lot at Universal Studios. We saw some film crews at work.

We got to go into the old mansion where they shoot the TV show *The Munsters*. Inside, there was this life-size statue of Grandpa Munster, a cranky old vampire. He was seated, wearing a skull cap with wires running to it, like he was being electrocuted. His hair stuck out from the sides of his head like wings and his nose and chin almost touched. My dad took a picture of me sitting on Grandpa Munster's lap. I'm really skinny and can barely sit up. My arms and legs are all taut and tangled. I look scared and very uncomfortable.

I was.

I will never forget the guy with the steel-gray eyes. Cruelty isn't something you see in a person's eyes, it's something you don't see. There's something missing. That guy looked at me the way people look at a frog splayed out in a specimen tray, prepped for dissection. He had no idea how to help me and didn't want to, anyway.

The memory of that day has faded, but there will always be a scar there. I did not realize then that my brush with torture would one day turn my silver pen into a sword.

9

THE HOUSE OF TOOTHPICKS

Withstanding the Surgical "Solution"

1964

Beatlemania grips America.

~

THE CHECKLIST IS complete. I am cleared for brain surgery.

I'm beginning to think that brain surgery could be what they do when they don't know what else to do. Maybe it's a sort of medical "Hail Mary," where the quarterback just throws the football as far as he can and hopes there's someone there to catch it.

I do not find this thought reassuring.

~

I'm at the UCLA Medical Center, near Grauman's Chinese Theater.

I'm in a bed in a hospital ward, just before the operation. In the bed straight across from me is a boy with freckles, a little younger than me. He's wearing blue pajamas and a white football helmet. I think he just had the same surgery that I'm going to have. He is sitting up, looking right at me. He says, "It's all right. It's all right to look at me."

He keeps on looking at me: freckles, pajamas, football helmet, and all. He is the first person I have ever seen who is so much like me. Looking at him makes me feel my own difference more sharply.

I look away.

I am on an operating table, my freshly shaved head in a big vise. It's so my head doesn't move during the surgery. The medical team put four screws into my skull so they could attach my head to the big metal frame that holds the vice.

The pain from the screws is excruciating. My body flops around like a fish on a dock. I tell my muscles to be still, but they don't listen to me. They are more rebellious than they've ever been before, as though they know what the surgery is for. The medical team can't knock me out because I have to be awake to help the surgeon figure out if the needle is in the right part of my brain. And during the surgery, I can't be allowed to move at all.

So they strap me down. My arms. My legs. My torso.

Then they put a needle in my arm. An I.V. But they do it wrong. They miss the vein and hit a nerve. They have to do it again.

I can't move any part of my body except my eyes. There are mirrors around on the walls and I can see some of what's going on. Doctors and nurses are moving around. They are all wearing masks. Bright lights. Lots of gleaming stainless-steel equipment with colored lights everywhere. Click. Buzz. Clink. Hum. Like a swarm of metallic insects. The paint they used to mark up my head for the incision smells ghastly. They drill a hole into my head.

When they put the needle into my head, it doesn't hurt. The nerves inside your brain don't feel pain. But the screws hurt. And the straps hurt.

And I can't move. And strangers wearing masks have drilled a hole into my skull and right now they are putting a giant needle into my brain!

I'm trapped in a nightmare, and I can't wake up.

They ask me lots of questions. Talking through their masks. "Can you count to ten, Neil?"

I count.

Then, "Count backwards from ten, Neil."

I count backwards.

They tell me to move my right hand, then my left foot. Then my fingers. "How about now?" A pause. "And now?"

After the surgery, I have to stay in bed. I'm in a hospital room, alone now. In fact, I don't think there's anyone else in this whole wing of the hospital. Footsteps echo. It sounds empty.

My dad brings me a tube of Duco Cement and a box of toothpicks. I build toothpick structures. The glue dries fast.

The next day, the surgeon comes in with another doctor and asks me to get out of bed and try to walk. He holds my arm in case I start to fall. It turns out I can walk pretty well, compared to before the surgery, anyway. I have to hold on to his arm to keep my balance, but still, this is good.

In the afternoon, my brother Russell, who is going to film school at USC, brings me a whole bunch of film cuttings, strips of celluloid left over from students editing their own films. He brought me a splicer so I can tape them together in unexpected combinations.

The following morning, the surgeon comes back to see how things are going. I get out of bed and walk, leaning on his arm. I don't do as well as the first time, but it's still better than before the surgery.

❧

My parents take me home, and for a while, my walking stays about the same. Then it gets a little better, then worse. And worse. And then it stays that way.

I spend a lot of time at home. It is a beautiful house on a hill in one of the best places to live in all the world. But it feels like a prison. Visitors are allowed.

For years, every Wednesday night, my parents have hosted a poker game around the big table in our living room. Drinks are served, and chips with dip. A lot of the people around the table are in the movie business, many of them writers.

Long ago, on one of the poker nights, before I went to summer camp, back when I could still walk, I was waiting outside the house next to the circular driveway, so I could watch the poker players arrive. I stood in the shadows by the front door to be semi-hidden, because of my limp. It was already getting dark when I heard a car coming up the driveway, a little too fast. My mom had told me there was a new guy coming that night. I thought this might be him. Yup. It was an older guy in a flashy white Alfa Romeo convertible. The wheels spat gravel. I'd never seen a car like that up close before.

After he parked, he got out, dropped his cigarette in the driveway and stepped on it, twisting his foot a little. Shiny white loafers. A suit the color of vanilla ice cream. He looked tired, maybe unhappy. Then he saw me by the front door and his whole face changed. He flashed me this big smile as he strode over, hand out. All tan and teeth.

"Hi, there! Is this the big game?"

I stepped toward him. His hair was meticulously styled and had exactly the right amount of silver running through it. He wore rings on his fingers as though he was some kind of Arabian prince. Even though he was being friendly, somehow I felt out of place, right there in my own driveway. This man looked a bit like Elvis. I shifted my weight as I put my hand out.

"Yeah."

We shook hands. He didn't notice my limp. I opened the door for him.

"Mike! Hail the conquering hero!"

Michael Wilson had just returned from France. He'd had to live and work there for a long time because he's a screenwriter and the studios in this country had blacklisted him. While in France, he had written the screenplay for the movie *Lawrence of Arabia*. It won the Oscar for Best Picture.

Last night, when Mike came through the front door, he was different. During a minor surgery, he'd had a stroke. He was sort of dragging one foot and slurring his words.

All the other players smiled and greeted Mike as he came to the table, the way they had on other nights.

"There he is! *Bon soir, mon ami!*"

"Hey, Mike!"

But the smiles on their faces as they greeted him seemed to be held in place by slightly different muscles than their usual smiles.

Mike's wife, Zelma, was with him. She looked a little nervous. He looked a bit fatter. She was trying to be cheerful. His face was sort of slack. She was acting like everything was just fine. He was wearing a bib. She was laughing. He seemed to have become a big baby. She was helping him with his food, his cards. Some dip dripped on his bib and then into his lap. Oh, God. She was joking around.

"Keep your eyes on your own cards, buster! Ha, ha, ha!"

Everybody was trying to help him, trying to be helpful. Telling jokes. Trying to kid around with him.

"Hey, Mike, don't win all the money. Leave a little for us! Ha, ha!"

In the kitchen, people were speaking in hushed tones. Eyes darting around. I couldn't hear what they were saying exactly, but I'm pretty sure it was about him.

Mike was trying to be upbeat, too. But life is much harder for him now. I could see that. He feels different now. I think he feels bad. I wonder what Mike thought of me now, sitting off to one side in my wheelchair.

I went to my room and thought about Mike.

And what it means to be different.

~

It is summer.

I spend a lot of time reading now, mostly comic books. I don't think my mom's too happy about that. Roger has lots of comic books that he keeps in a box in the back of his closet. Years ago, he gave me my first comic. It was *Green Lantern*, a DC comic. I still like *Green Lantern* comic books. To me, a green lantern is the perfect symbol of power and triumph. I need that now.

Roger recently brought me a couple of his newer ones. We sat on my bed and flipped through them together.

"They have all these new superheroes! They're from Marvel! They're really neat!"

He started reading one of them out loud, giving each character a different voice, the way he does when he makes up funny stories at the dinner table. He's really good at it. I started giggling and pretty soon he cracked up, too.

Roger is right. They are neat. Really neat.

I want the rest of them. While the little drugstore in Ojai has a comic book rack, it doesn't have much of a selection. Besides, I'd have to go in there all the time to get the new issues. When I went to Santa Barbara with my parents, I saw the comic book racks inside a big drugstore from the back seat of the car. They have a lot more comics than they have in Ojai, but I'm not going in there. It would be too hard and too public. My parents would probably do it for me, but I don't think they'd really approve. And what about getting new issues? I thought of writing a letter to the store owner, detailing the location of the comic racks, listing the names and numbers of the issues I wanted to buy, explaining my "situation" and asking him to mail them to me. I thought about asking my dad to deliver the letter for me. Or maybe Roger.

My favorite Marvel superhero is Professor X, leader of the mutant superhero group The X-men. He is a genius with the power to both read and control the minds of others. The X-Men protect mutants and fight against injustice. And Professor X can't walk. He uses a wheelchair. But it's no big deal. It's not even an important part of the story. Amazing.

It is July. Today, the latest Marvel comic came in the mail. Addressed to me. It just miraculously appeared. Somebody bought me a subscription. Roger? Dad? Mom?

～

It's been almost a year now, and I'm about the same as I was before the surgery. I am getting skinnier, though. Can't eat. This is not good.

The doctors say they may have frozen the wrong cells and would like to give it another try. They want to take another crack at me.

Deep breath. Round two.

Here goes.

IO
Late-Night TV
Medical Rematch

1965

The Age of Aquarius dawns.

~

I'M BACK AT THE UCLA Medical Center, but in a different part of it. In a big room with high ceilings and plaster walls. I'm on my back in a gurney, a bed with side railings and wheels, looking at the skylight. The room is chilly.

A surgeon steps into view. He looks at me in a friendly way and asks, "Which would be more important to you, Neil: walking, or speaking?"

I am ten years old now. An image of me hiking on a sunlit mountainside pops unbidden into my head, and, in a rush to a decision, I answer.

"Walking."

The surgery seems to take days.

Pain slows down time. So does fear.

~

After the surgery, I have my own hospital room. Just like last time, but with a TV. I stay up way past my bedtime and watch shows they won't let me see at home. I even see *One Step Beyond*.

This surgery didn't work any better than the first. Even though I can walk a little better, there's no improvement in my other movements and I can barely eat at all. Swallowing is really hard. I guess maybe they froze the wrong brain cells again.

I spend a lot of my time practicing using my new body. It isn't easy learning what I can do and how I can do it.

Speech is very difficult now. They give me a "word board." It is like a Ouija board, but things are written on it like "yes," "no," and "okay." I add, "Corned beef hash, please," and, "Want to play poker?" I wonder if my answer to the surgeon about walking was right. Maybe not.

I talk less now. I am usually in the shadows off to the side of any group, keenly aware that I may be made fun of at any minute. Not that anyone actually makes fun of me, but I am always on my guard. I use words sparingly, reluctantly, as tools to accomplish specific tasks.

Once home, I look for things to do that don't require a lot of walking and talking. I settle on bocce ball. When Mike Wilson was in France, he had taken up bocce ball. Now he comes over to our place to play. He's still recovering from his stroke, so it's a good activity for him. Not too strenuous. We are well matched.

Under the normal rules, a ball is thrown from a distance, underhand, palm down. Mike and I tacitly agree that this is pointlessly restrictive and explore more practical techniques. Mike is perfecting what I call the "double-handed drop," often executed directly above the target area, like a bomber. It is effective. One of my techniques involves lowering myself to all fours in order to adjust the position of the balls with my hand. It is very effective.

What Mike has become scares me. He is a victim, an unimportant member of society. Who would go to him now for help with anything? He is helpless. Now he wears a onesie, a one-piece suit, because it's easy for him to put on and take off. He's a huge baby now, who wears a bib.

I cannot let that happen to me.

~

It's been a year, and the doctors say they want to give it one more try, this time in New York with a famous surgeon. I tell Roger that it's two pitches, two strikes. Two failed brain surgeries.

Roger says, "Maybe three's a charm."

I I

HORSESHOES

Yet Another Brain Freeze

September 1966
Star Trek debuts.

~

I am scrunched up on the back seat of a taxi, all knees and elbows, sweating. My dad is in front with his arm out the window, talking with the driver, glancing back after every block. Smelly bus exhaust drifts in with the sounds of traffic. We are lost in a sea of cars and boulevards, between tall buildings of brick and stone.

We pull up to a red brick hospital in a poor neighborhood in the Bronx, about fifteen miles south of our old house in Scarsdale. The hospital used to be called "Home for the Incurables," which seems pretty bleak. Now it's called "St. Barnabas," which sounds a little better.

In admissions, they write down my current condition, before the surgery. Pre-op.

"Patient is 11. He is almost totally immobilized. He can crawl on all fours, but only for a few feet. He can't keep his head up off his chest. He is hardly able to swallow anything. His weight has dropped from 93 to 62 pounds since his last surgery. He is emaciated."

For a while now, I have been eating most of my meals through a straw. My constantly flexed muscles and tendons burn a lot of calories. I am just skin and bones.

In the surgeon's office, I meet the secretary, Joan. When she was a child, the surgeon performed this same procedure on her. It worked. I don't talk to her, but I watch her. She walks around like there's nothing to it. I am so impressed that she has lived what I am going through. I feel like she really understands. I think of her as a goddess, like Aphrodite. She gives me courage.

I meet my new surgeon, Dr. Irving S. Cooper, the pioneer of freezing brain cells with needles. Many years ago, someone gave him a bottle opener that shot cold carbon dioxide through a needle to pop corks off wine bottles. He said, "Eureka!" Then he invented cryothalamotomies.

Dr. Cooper is the champion who will do battle with my rebel brain cells. He's done more of these procedures with a higher rate of success than anyone else in the world. There are pictures in a magazine of him playing paddle tennis at his home in New Jersey. He's wearing white shorts. It says he has a white schnauzer named Odin. Dr. Cooper is the best. But I'm still scared.

I'm on the operating table. I've already been here for hours. Dr. Cooper is poking the needle into my head right now trying to decide when to turn on the liquid nitrogen. He asks me to speak many times, to check to see which cells the needle is touching. "Say the letters of the alphabet, Neil."

I have to be patient. "A.B.C."

A while later he asks, "Can you move the fingers of your left hand, Neil?" I'm very hot and sweating heavily, very uncomfortable. A voice says,

"Minus 60 degrees." I feel a rush of cool air as a nurse lifts the sheet off my feet. I think she noticed my discomfort. I smile.

"Open your left hand, Neil," says Dr. Cooper.

My left hand unclenches slowly, like a flower blooming.

The surgery was a week ago.

I am in a brightly lit lecture hall filled with men in long white lab coats. Standing at the center of the stage, looking up at them, is Dr. Cooper, also in a white lab coat. He is the king here. The others defer to him, the master of the cryothalamotomy.

I am on the stage, too. On one side of me is Dr. Cooper, on the other, my wheelchair.

That's right.

I am standing on the stage.

I can use my left side again.

It's like I'm back at the helm and a breeze is filling my sails. Or at least one sail. My left hand and my left foot are back under my control. Not completely, but a lot more than they were before the surgery. And I can pick up my head from my chest.

While it is true that most of my weight is on my left leg, I'm not leaning on anything. It's also true that I'm not standing ramrod straight. And, yes, my right arm is more or less locked at a ninety-degree angle. And, yes, I am in my underwear.

But.

I am standing.

This alone is front page news.

This simple act is an event of such importance that *Life* magazine has sent a reporter to record it. He asks me a couple of questions and writes my answers down in his notepad. My dad stands next to him, beaming.

Not only can I stand, but my speech is a bit clearer, and I can chew better and swallow more easily, too. Now I can eat more and put some meat on these bones.

It's not perfect, but it's definitely better.

And better is good.

I've got my own hospital room. A candy-striper with a ponytail named Jenny takes me to a tiny cafe down in a corner of the hospital's basement. It doesn't seem very promising, but turns out to serve fantastic tomato sandwiches. Fresh rye bread with a spread of mayo. Jenny calls me her boyfriend.

In a way, a cyrothalamotomy is like horseshoes.

Close counts.

❧

When I get out of the hospital, my dad and I go to stay at my uncle's place outside the city. I have to go see Dr. Cooper a few times so he can see how I'm doing. Post-op follow-up.

I watch a lot of TV at my uncle's house. There's a new show called *Star Trek* with a character named Christopher Pike. He had been the captain of a starship and was severely injured while trying to rescue his crew. He uses a wheelchair-like vehicle that looks like a big box that only his head sticks out of. He can't walk or talk, but he can control the chair's movements with his brainwaves. He communicates by means of a small light bulb on the front of the box. One blink means "yes," two blinks means "no." That's pretty much it. The captain of the starship Enterprise, James T. Kirk, defers to Pike, and not just because of his rank.

My cousin's ex-husband, Gregory Massell, came to my uncle's Christmas party. As he sat down beside me on the floor, he groaned, smiled, and said, "Sore back." Then he told me about surviving the winter in a Siberian prison camp. He told me it got so cold that the horses died. I found this story oddly comforting, probably because an adult was telling me something that was real. For several years now, most of what I have been hearing from adults is fairy tales with happy endings.

~

I'm back home and my dad's old friend, Dan, came to visit us. He won an Oscar for writing the screenplay for *From Here to Eternity*. He brought me three records. *The Monkees, Mary Poppins*, and the new one by Petula Clark. I fashion a drum set out of old Folgers cans with snap-on lids and play along with "Downtown." Just being able to do this is great.

My speech really is better, but people still have a hard time understanding me. And I'm still scared to talk to people. I can tell how uncomfortable it makes them. And now my eyebrows, which have always loyally followed my silent orders, have decided to join the rebel forces. They start raising and lowering themselves whenever they want. These movements distract people who are trying to understand me. I see this eyebrow insurrection as a new low.

On Wednesday nights, though, I talk with the poker players in our living room. One of the writers for the *Batman* TV show asks me about when I write. He asks me if I hear the words in my head before I write them. I tell him I do. And then I think, "Who am I? What do I have to say?" And I listen to the voice in my head that asked those questions and realize that, unlike my speech, that voice is very clear.

I've never had thoughts like this before.

50

12

I Can Walk

Hopes and Dreams

Early 1967

Flower power is in full bloom.

Planet of the Apes is in production. Screenplay by Rod Serling and
Mike Wilson.

I'VE BEEN BACK IN Ojai for about six months now, going to the same
school as before.

I'm not a kid anymore. I'm 13, and in the ninth grade.

Yes, I'm a little young to be in ninth grade, but I've always been on the
honor roll, and I'm pretty good at schoolwork. When my parents asked me
if I wanted to skip a grade, I said, "Why not?"

The classes are a bit more interesting. While I have learned how to
diagram compound-complex sentences, I don't know why. Algebra seems
pointless, too. Taking tests is tedious. On the other hand, I am being introduced to some wonderful poetry. I'm writing more of my own.

A guy at school named Robert starts calling me "Herbivorous." It's like his code word for strange. He's not really doing it to be mean. He teases other guys, too, gives them nicknames, and so on. All the guys tease each other. Like bear cubs wrestling. But my nickname is different, somehow. The word spreads and all the kids are talking about it. Some of the girls are shocked, as though a taboo has been broken.

In an odd way, when Robert calls me Herbivorous, there's a certain raw honesty to it. He is smart, popular, and feared. It could be that he's picking on me because if he didn't, he wouldn't be fulfilling his sacred obligation to pick on everyone. I think he sees himself as an equal-opportunity bully. Besides, it's better than being treated with kid gloves all the time. I am learning that there's such a thing as too much "nice." In a way, if Robert wanted to be a really fair bully, he would call me something worse, like "Limp Gimp." Something with a little more sting.

～

Okay. Something good is happening.

My right foot, which has stayed arched and pointed inward for the last several years, is straightening out. I can stand on it. The toe still wants to point inward, but the tug is weaker every day.

After a month, suddenly, both of my legs work. My feet are more or less straight. Almost no tugging. My gait is still different from other people's, but I really am walking. Almost like there's nothing to it.

Soon, I am taking long walks, then hikes. I can ride a bike again. And go surfing.

After Dr. Cooper's surgery, my left side was better, but now, both sides are better. Not perfect, but really better. For some reason, my legs have improved much more than my arms and hands.

The doctors call it remission. They say, "Spontaneous remissions are often temporary." That means it probably won't last very long. They say, "To be frank with you, Neil…." "Frank" doesn't mean anything.

I don't dare hope that this dramatic improvement will last, the way it did for Joan. I just can't. But, here's the thing: I can't not hope, either. I can't.

⌒

Francesca is my Spanish teacher. She is from Spain. She speaks with us as equals, as friends. Words and language are poetry to her. Life is philosophy. She enjoys telling us about real life.

When she was a girl, she met the artist Salvador Dali in a field behind her house. She showed us a picture of one of his paintings. It was of boiled beans all twisted together to make them look like a person in torment.

Every day in Francesca's class, we have to write a paragraph in Spanish. I always write a poem instead. The subject of my daily poem is always the same. Love. And, although I don't think she knows it, the poem is always about her.

Together, Francesca and I go to a movie in town. On the way there, I am nervous. You know how people say that teenagers feel self-conscious about how their bodies are different? Well, that's not quite the same thing. I mean, my body really is different. Yes, I can walk now, but my body still isn't lined up straight, so the way I walk is different. And my speech is still slow and hard to understand. So it's hard for me to be out in public, to be on display. It's like I've been put in the stocks in the town square.

We're outside the theater, standing in line under the marquee. It's a warm evening in early summer and I feel people watching me. I feel them judging me. I just want to hide. This is almost unbearable. Then Francesca leans toward me and quietly says, "Going out with you, I feel a little bit like royalty, with the way people are looking at us."

That is perhaps the best thing that anyone has ever said to me.

In Ojai, my mom is known as "the actress." The other actress in town is her friend, Liz.

Liz is tall and lanky, with a low, hoarse smoker's voice and a long scarf. She always wears a brightly colored hat with a huge floppy brim. Her green eyes stick out from under heavy, dark lashes. Her hair is thick and black and her skin is leathery from sun and tobacco.

Whenever Liz enters a room, it's as though she's saying, "Yes, I know … and?" She is defiant. "What are you looking at?" No subject is small, in Liz's eyes. But she has no use for small talk, either. She has no fear of truth. She thumbs her nose at convention. Always unpredictable, never playing by the rules.

It's as if there's always a camera following her around. She's always on. Always a star, burning bright. Always performing. Whether the audience can see, hear, or appreciate her doesn't matter. Liz is playing the beautiful hostess to a fabulous world. She says "darling" all the time.

I'm uneasy around her. I may have to see and feel things in a new way. I might get hurt.

At a party one night at a neighbor's house, I'm sitting off to one side, alone, bored, and without hope. I want to go somewhere, but I have nowhere to go. I'm so self-absorbed, I'm barely functioning. I can't see outside myself.

Liz walks over to me and gives me a wide, knowing smile.

"Darling. Let's dance."

The stage is set. I am ready for whatever has brought us here.

I'm thrilled. I realize that I've been waiting for just this moment. We go out on the floor and without a word, I become Astaire, she becomes Ginger. Her gaze meets mine. Then we assume the posture of high romance, cheek to cheek. Out here, dancing with Liz, I feel pride. I feel a sense of completeness and power that I haven't felt before.

This isn't a dance scene from some musical. It is a rite of passage.

For the first time, I glimpse the world of limitless possibility. Liz showed it to me.

Now I have dreams, places to go. I want to live on a hilltop and sleep under the stars. I want to stare at the night sky and wonder at its measureless depths. I want to travel across rolling hills and live a life of adventure and love that is as beautiful and sensual as morning fog lit by glowing moons and dawning suns. I want to live in a world of skateboards and surfboards and motorbikes. I want to go on tour with Country Joe and the Fish. We'll go around the world and spread the message of love to help save this world! We will sing and laugh and dance! I can get there from here.

I'm no longer a child. I am now aware of the kind of love that is super-charged by sensual attraction. I understand my friend's fascination with the lingerie section of the Sears catalog. As things are right now, with my body working as well as it is, I eagerly anticipate having a girlfriend, going steady, and falling in love. I see myself as a romantic kind of guy, sensitive to soft hands, warm skin, and the scent of girls. I feel embraceable, ready to accept, and to give love.

I'm about to start tenth grade. It's clear to me that because of my surgeries and all the time I was using a wheelchair my childhood was really sheltered. I have some catching up to do.

I tell my parents that it would be better for me to be more independent. They agree with me, and I move into the boys' dorms on the hill above the school. My dorm room is like a rustic cabin that overlooks a wild canyon, thick with oak and acacia. Outside my window, the fog rolls in from the coast most mornings and fills the valley and its side canyons with a veil of mist that vanishes before noon.

In 1937, Frank Capra made *Lost Horizons*, a film about a valley called Shangri-La, hidden somewhere in the mountains of Asia. It is an earthly paradise, breathtakingly beautiful, where people live for centuries, aging gracefully without suffering. As the shooting location for Shangri-La, Capra chose the Ojai Valley.

In this close-knit community of boarding students, I read poetry and learn about philosophy. In a way, I'm a monk in a monastery.

I guess you could say I'm living in paradise. At least for now.

13

A Message in a Bottle

A Moment of Doubt and Pain

Late fall 1968

Martin Luther King was assassinated in April.

Robert Kennedy was assassinated in June.

Half million American soldiers are fighting in Vietnam.

I AM FOURTEEN.

It has been hard for me to speak for a long time. All of the muscles I use to speak are hard to control, but my tongue is the worst. Often, when I am about to speak, I open my mouth wide and my tongue goes in and out three or four times, as though it's warming up for the task ahead. My vocal cords will sometimes start up before they are needed, like a jet revving its engines before take-off. Then I bring my jaw and lip muscles into play, jockeying them into position for the word I'm about to say. Most people's speech muscles work together like a team of Chinese acrobats, standing on each others' shoulders and spinning plates on sticks, all while riding on the same bicycle. Like there's nothing to it. My vocal acrobats lack teamwork.

When I talk, it is slow, halting, and very strained. It sounds like a recording of a drowning chipmunk slowed down about ten times. But no. Maybe a baby water buffalo mired in quicksand. But that's not it, either, because the tone of my voice is very smooth and low. I have a great sense of pitch, too. It's the pronunciation of the words that's wrong, not the pitch or the tone. I actually have a great voice.

Even now, during this remission, when I speak, I have to pare the message down to the fewest syllables possible. Imagine that your sole means of communication is stamping out a message in the snow that can only be read from a plane that passes overhead once each day. Imagine that sometimes the plane doesn't show up. It feels like that. Sometimes I just give up.

I end up saying simple things. Like "yes," or "no," or "I can't say." One I use a lot is, "It's a long story." Another thing that is very easy for me to say is "garbanzo beans." Sadly, the subject rarely comes up.

I've been walking everywhere for several months now. With only a slight limp. Although I'm still uncomfortable walking in public and I still long for open highways and endless summers, I find that beaches are quite wonderful, as are frisbees and sting-ray bikes with tall handle bars.

It's summer. A friend who lives on a ranch in a canyon invites me over. My dog, Wy-mar, comes with me. We pack two knapsacks with a map, a compass, water, and sack lunches that my friend's mom made for us. His mom is great. There's no BS with her. And no pity.

We hike into the mountains behind the ranch. It is hot. After hiking up a narrow valley for a couple of hours, we sit facing a jagged cliff where water falls right in front of us as we munch our pastrami sandwiches. I give Wy-mar two chunks. We are tired and smiling, cooled by the drifting mist.

We start back. It is easier going down the valley.

What's this? My right foot is turning inward again. My gait changes. If it keeps on doing this, if it gets worse, I won't be able to put my weight on it.

My mind asks, "Is this me? What's wrong? Am *I* doing this?" My thoughts are confused.

The tug gets stronger, and my foot becomes that familiar crescent. Walking suddenly becomes difficult.

I stumble. Wy-mar gives me a worried look.

My friend has been watching. He asks, "Do you want me to carry you?"

I answer, "No." I don't want to be carried.

Is this a dream? Will I wake up? Will it go away?

This isn't good at all. Walking is suddenly very hard again.

I keep going. It's hard to do, but I do it. I finish the hike.

❧

It's fall. A new school year starts. Living at school. With a roommate, but on my own.

I'm scared. Thousands of men are being drafted into the army. What if they draft Roger? What if they send him to Vietnam? What if they send me? At a dinner party, I sit crying at the dinner table and write a note to President Nixon asking him not to do that. Not to draft Roger. And not me. My mom helps me send it. I never got an answer.

Okay. This is bad. My right foot has turned in again. And my right leg is becoming completely insubordinate, doing its own thing.

To help me get around campus, my parents buy me a used golf cart. It's pretty beat up, but at least it's better than that clunky old wheelchair.

Now I can hardly walk. Mostly, I have to hop, using my left leg, because my right leg sticks straight out, like I just kicked a field goal. My right hand once again makes a tight fist, and my right shoulder spasms are severe and almost continuous, throwing me off balance. My torso is twisted, and my arms and hands are very hard to control.

The remission is over.

⌐

Staring out the window of my dorm room with tears in my eyes. I am in pain. Not physical pain, but the pain of loneliness, of separation. And I am mad at myself for being in pain. I don't know who else or what else to be mad at. Who else is there to blame? Should I yell at God? I think of running away. But I can't run, of course. The bottom of the hill is about as far as I'd get.

I go outside my dorm room. It is quite early. I slowly make my way along a dirt path to a break in a row of eucalyptus trees. Hopping, swinging one leg. The mist is disappearing with the morning sunlight. I stop and turn toward the valley below. As the day warms up, a few flies gather in the sunbeams, each in a little holding pattern, drawing random circles of flight. Time slows.

I hear questions that I don't want to hear. Putting my fingers in my ears wouldn't do any good. The questions are coming from inside my head.

"What do you have to give?"

"Nothing," I answer.

"What are you worth?"

"Nothing," I answer.

"Who are you?"

"No one."

And then come accusations.

"You are unlovable. No one will ever love you. You are too ugly. Too grotesque. And you can't love. You can't even reach out to anyone. No one understands you. No one ever will. There will be no girlfriend, no wife, no happy family. There will be no love. Face it, you have no future. Why don't you just give up!"

And there, on the ground next to my left foot, I see a piece of green broken glass. It is as though someone placed it there, just for me. Will this stop the aching in my heart?

I pick up the shard of glass and cut my right wrist.

All of the fear, shame, doubt, and pain; all the loneliness and self-loathing pours out of me. Much of what has been hidden, trapped, and building up pressure inside me is now erupting. My heart bursts open. I sit there, crying. In that moment of release, I realize that at the center of all this turmoil is love: having it, giving it, feeling it, sharing it, accepting it. The only answer to the accusing voice is love. I also understand that I need help, that I have needed help, and that help is nearer now that my pain has been made visible.

As fast as I can, I head back to the dorms, one leg hopping, one swinging, to the room of a friend I trust. He wraps my wrist in white towels. As I sit in his room sobbing, he asks me if it's okay to call a teacher. I say yes, and the teacher arrives, breathless. Still crying, I tell them how tired I am of the mundane tasks and struggle of everyday life, how hard it is just to be me. I tell them that I have nowhere to go. I tell them I have no hope.

I didn't understand what was happening to me.

In my early teens, I had dreams of a future full of love and happiness. Today, I know that every teenager has such dreams. It is what teenagers do, what they should do. And when those dreams suddenly seem unattainable, it is not unusual for a teenager to despair. When the remission ended, it became harder for me to imagine any bright future that had me in it. All I had was an old golf cart. Now, it could have become harder anyway, even if the remission had continued. I don't know. Probably no one knows.

Think of it this way, I had been standing on the top of a hill. Stretched out below me was a land of beauty and love. Then, instead of getting closer, that waiting land seemed to be moving farther and farther away. It made my heart ache. And I thought I was supposed to have control over my own heart. So I thought it was my fault.

I didn't know then how much of my pain was caused by our society's bizarre expectations of what it then called, and still calls, disability. I didn't really know about our society's problems dealing with the differences between human beings. So, I blamed myself, and the voice of self-doubt and self-loathing became, in that moment, very persuasive.

The teacher says, "I'd like to call your folks, Neil. Is that okay?"

Through my tears, again I say yes. The teacher cleans and tightly bandages my wrist. By the time my parents come into the dorm room, I'm in bed, resting. I keep my eyes closed as they come over to me. They don't know that I'm awake.

Now they are looking at my wrist, talking in whispers. I continue to pretend to be asleep. I still don't know how to explain myself to them. How do you explain to your parents, or to anybody, that the world needs to be transformed by the pain that pushes you to love?

⌁

I wake up in the dark.

I'm at home, in my own bedroom. My wrist is bound in fresh white bandages. The door has been left half-opened, a night light in the hall left on. I hear muted voices. As quietly as I can, I get out of bed and make my way over to the door. Leaning against the wall, I look out, careful to stay within the darkness of my room. Across the hall and down a bit, the door to my parents room has been left half-opened as well. Through it, I can see my mom and dad sitting on the bed, her hand on his shoulder. The reading light from the bedside table illuminates their faces from the side and below, making sharp ridges of light and valleys of shadow. I have never seen them look like this before.

My dad is hunched forward, elbows on knees, hands clasped tightly, shoulders gently shaking.

"I've failed my son," he sobs, his face contorted. "I failed him."

"That's not true," my mom says.

I feel bad for him, but I don't know what he's talking about. Why would he think that it's his fault?

Pain is pain.

What can I do?

14
EMBRACEABLE ME
The Life-Changing Power of Love

Summer 1969

Jimi Hendrix will play "The Star-Spangled Banner" at Woodstock.

Neil Armstrong will walk on the moon.

∽

I'M STILL 15.

My dad has a friend in Seattle named Harvey who's been developing a method of helping people called re-evaluation co-counseling. When my dad suggests we go see Harvey, right away I say, "Okay."

∽

The counseling center is a casual, homey place, full of books, throw rugs, and overstuffed sofas. Compared to the noise and bustle of the downtown Seattle streets below, the center feels like an oasis of peaceful flexibility in a rigid, contentious world.

Every night, Harvey tells stories that show how people are naturally good. We're all born that way, and we then get hurt by other people and by society. He explains how that original, natural goodness gets obscured by the pain of those experiences.

Some of his stories are about adults who get stressed and yell at their children. These external put-downs become the mantras that the children silently say to themselves over and over as they become adults.

"I'm sorry. I'm the problem. It's my fault. I can't do anything right. I'm just in the way. Don't pay any attention to me. I'm worthless. I'm nobody."

The noise of these mantras can drown out the clear voice of innate goodness and limit potential and the ability to accept and to give love.

Harvey's stories make sense to me. They help me make sense of the world.

Most of the people here are around 40. Many of them have been abused and neglected. And they've overcome those problems and climbed up out of their old lives. It's like they've remade themselves into something stronger.

I see that the women here are in leadership roles in a way that I haven't seen elsewhere. Maybe it's because it's easier for them to show their emotions and to talk about feelings than it is for the men.

The center is full of people sitting in pairs. All the people are learning how to really listen to each other, to find out where each other's old hurts are, so that those hurts can be brought out into the open. When the pain of those hurts is discharged, the innate goodness of that person can re-emerge and they can realize their full potential.

Several times, Harvey is my co-counselor. He knows exactly which questions to ask. He is very busy, though, so most of the time I work with other people.

I am sitting on the floor across from my counselor, Michelle. I start to explain what's going on with me. Like many of the younger women at the center, she has long straight brown hair, parted down the center. Her eyes are green, serene, and set far apart. Slowly, with great care and effort, I speak.

"My. Problem. Is. With. Love." I can tell she is having trouble under-standing me. I try again.

"It's. About. Love. And. Desire." Her face is what can only be described as blank. Serene, but blank. One more time.

"I. Am. Confused," but, I realize, not as confused as she is. So far, this session doesn't seem to be helping me all that much.

Over Michelle's shoulder, I see a woman approaching. She is so beautiful. She's like a mirage. She smiles softly and gestures for me not to worry, as if she is reassuring someone locked up in a cage. She says her name is Colleen. To me, she seems like a goddess, and I am intimidated. I want to be respectful, the way a mortal should be in the presence of a goddess. I see myself reflected in her beauty and grace. But her long, smooth, womanly legs keep distracting me. I find it hard to believe that she is even talking to me.

Colleen says she has an idea that she thinks might help me. She sits down in front of me and tells me to relax.

Okay. Here I am, pretending to relax. There's certainly nowhere to hide now.

Then she leans forward and very matter-of-factly hugs me and starts kissing me.

It is like a waking dream.

I know that it sounds strange, but I feel as though I have been seen, really seen, for the first time. She has caught me completely by surprise. What's going on here? It's like I'm not invisible anymore. Not only that, but until today, I've never understood what people meant when they said they were comfortable in their own skin. I mean, in her eyes, I am her equal. Colleen saw what many others had missed: this young man needs loving. Her kisses, her hugs, her laugh. I don't know. She woke me up. She really did. Like sunrise.

⌒

Many years later, I was being interviewed on a talk show and the interviewer asked me if I could recall a particular moment in my life when I had developed my positive self-image. And, flash! There was the answer: a kiss! So simple. So true.

~

My dad and I fly home. I look at him asleep in the seat beside me.

I've only been gone a week, but I feel different about myself. I realize now that my blue eyes are bright and beautiful. I realize now that, far from being grotesque, I am handsome. For the first time, I know what it feels to be worth something. And in my belly and in my heart, there is a fire that leaps out into my life, into the lives of the people around me, and into my writing.

I decide to write something every day.

~

It's still summer. My sister Kendra invites me to visit her in Berkeley. Her boyfriend drives us around in his MG. We have a picnic in the Berkeley Hills. At the campus theater we see *Dr. Strangelove*. After the show, we walk up and down Telegraph Avenue. On this warm summer evening, the counterculture is in full flower. The sidewalks are full of all kinds of people. A busker sings "Like a Rolling Stone" and a group of students join in the chorus. I feel very exposed, like I'm standing in front of the morning assembly again, trying to sing "Land of Hope and Glory." What should be a very cool experience for me is more like a form of torture. I have to get past this shame. "*How does it feeeeel?*"

The next day, we drive up to my cousin Nina's place in Mill Valley, a glass house with a warm kitchen set in a redwood forest under starry skies. Nina and her children are living poetic lives and thinking very deep thoughts.

Lots of stories. I just watch them. I take it all in. Nina speaks to me as if she understands it all already. She makes me feel very welcome.

I want to know how to deal with this. And flying kites, storytelling, and mail-order catalogs seem to help, as do collage and decoupage. I don't want to be ashamed of my difference. I don't want to hide anymore. I now know that I have the power to love and to be loved. I promise myself that I will use this power.

15

MUNCHKINLAND

Life in a Boarding School

1970

The Beatles broke up.

Nixon deploys American ground troops to northern Cambodia.

~

I AM 16, AND BACK AT boarding school.

About sixty boys live up here above the canyon. I'd like to say we're like the Lost Boys in Neverland, but we're not. It's more like we're a band of wayward kids whose parents have enough money to pay the tuition to send us here and, for whatever reason, pay it.

I'm in the same room as before, my eagle's nest, perched on the rim of the canyon. My golf cart is my chariot. I manipulate the controls with my left hand and steer with my right, giving other kids rides down the hill to class. I bomb around campus in it, like Apollo. Last year, they called me Herbivorous. Now, I am just Herb, or Herbie. Herbivorous is past. Forgotten.

I am now Herbie, a cool guy. I am in.

My classmates and I are keenly aware that the world outside our valley is changing, and we want to be part of it. The music that pours out of the dorm rooms and echoes down the valley declares our allegiance. Cream. Hendrix. Led Zeppelin. Drugs are on campus. The rumors about who is using what never stop. At night, the aroma of burning marijuana drifts down from the area up the canyon that we call "Munchkinland." In the sexual revolution, we have sided with the insurgents, if only as cheerleaders.

The school organizes a field trip to see *Easy Rider*. I hesitate, not really wanting to be in public, but I'm glad I went. We all identify with Peter Fonda and Dennis Hopper, heading out on the highway, looking for adventure. We're ready to jump the fence.

My history teacher is Mr. Higginbotham. He seems nice enough, but I think he's hiding something. I suspect he was born off-planet.

I raised my hand in his class, "Was. It. The. Romans. Who. Invented. Aqueducts?" I had no interest in either Romans or aqueducts. My labored question was intended as a test. It was a test of my power of speech, and of my ability to overcome my fear of speaking. It was also a test of my classmates' and teacher's ability to face their fear. It was an experiment in social power.

The guy who sits next to me in history wears very thick glasses. I think about Cyrano de Bergerac and about the hasty judgments that people make. Because I don't speak a lot, many people assume I'm thinking deep thoughts, and they ask what I'm thinking. I've noticed that people who are smart seem to believe I am, too, and that people who seem less so often jump to the conclusion that I am not too bright. In a way, I'm a mirror.

I do my homework on a typewriter. My teachers find it easier to read my typing than my handwriting. The most difficult part about typing is constantly having to feed in a fresh sheet of paper. Each time I do this, I am reminded that the designers of this machine were thinking of end users other than me.

I type with the index finger of my left hand. The whole process is slow, but it works. I have an understanding with my teachers that no points will be deducted for errors in spelling or punctuation. I have lots of love poems. A stack of them. I think I'll be a writer. I can write poetry, books, plays.

In accordance with the dress code, I wear a necktie. It's a clip-on. It works. Although my green bell-bottoms violate the code, no one says anything. Good thing, too, they're my only pants with Velcro.

I am comfortable living here. I have lots of freedom. I don't have to wait tables or wash dishes, and I can sit wherever I want at meals. These guys are my friends. They aren't shocked by my ways. They know how I walk, talk, and eat. They're used to me and I'm used to them. I don't feel like I have to hide from them. Sure, sometimes I feel a twinge of shame, or a bit of self-consciousness, but it's nothing like before. Instead of being hold-your-breath intolerable, it's something I can manage, and live with.

Not only that, but I've come to accept and like myself, and sometimes, even to love myself.

Dr. Cooper comes to the campus with my dad. Afterward, my dad tells me that he asked Dr. Cooper if another surgery might be a good idea. His answer?

"It would be too risky."

~

On a flight to visit Kendra, I'm seated next to Fess Parker, the guy who played Davy Crockett and Daniel Boone. I tell him that I'm going to be a writer.

"I'm. going. to. write. a play."

He smiles at me and says, "On opening night, I'll be there. Look for me in the front row. I'll be wearing a tuxedo."

~

The whole school goes on a field trip to the Renaissance Faire, a fake Medieval English market town filled with people in costume and in character. Think of Disney adding a low-budget Shakespeareland.

One of the booths sells kisses for a quarter. Some of the kids from the school buy one. I stand off to one side and pretend that I'm not watching. I think of Colleen and how a kiss can affect a person, how one affected me. I am both drawn to and terrified by this booth.

The other thing that grabs my attention is that I am in a crowd of people. They're not my classmates or my family, not people I know and who know me. They're strangers, but I'm actually looking them straight in the eye. And I'm noticing details of their appearance, like their glass love beads and the needlepoint in their denim jackets. A new sense of security allows me the freedom to notice small things like this. They're still watching me, of course. I'm not invisible. But here's the thing: while I still feel the urge to hide, I'm not in agony.

I even go up to a concession stand, reach into my pocket, take out my money, and buy a candied apple on a stick. The concessionaire hands it to me, with my change. I eat the candied apple. Right there. In public.

That probably doesn't sound like a big deal, but to me, it is a very big deal. Consider. A shiny-red candied apple on a stick is not something that can be eaten inconspicuously. The people around you will almost certainly notice. And if you are eating a candied apple and happen to have dystonia, well, they're going to notice.

Here I am, holding a half-eaten, shiny-red candied apple on the end of the stick. I am in the open, in broad daylight, in the warm California sun. Surrounded by strangers. Completely exposed. Chomping away, mouth wet and wide. I am doing this deliberately, bravely fighting back my shame with every bite. It is an act of will.

As I look around at all the people, it hits me hard how sheltered my life has been, how being ashamed of my difference has so thoroughly boxed me in. It sounds funny, but eating this bright red candied apple on a stick at Renaissance Faire is a personal triumph. It has opened my eyes. It has opened another world of possibility. It makes me want to face things full-on, things that, until now, I've only imagined facing.

I really must get out more.

16

TAKING THE REINS

A Valedictory Message

Early 1971
At UC Berkeley, the Disabled Students Program starts up.
Eric Clapton and Duane Allman play together on "Layla."

~

I'M A SENIOR NOW, and it's weird. Because I'm not hiding as much, scurrying around with my head down, I can see others much more clearly. And one thing that I've noticed is that my friends here are suffering. I used to think that my suffering, my pain, was caused by dystonia alone. I thought that all my problems would be well on their way to being solved if it would just go away.

But none of these kids needs a wheelchair. They all play lacrosse. I sit on the hill above the field and watch them. I'm the only one here who has earned the distinction of being called disabled.

And yet they suffer, too.

~

I'll graduate soon. My friends and I have these talks that go late into the night. We talk about things that teenage boys don't usually discuss. About our emotions, our feelings, our pain. It's probably because we'll be leaving soon that we're opening up so much. It may also have something to do with my counseling experience.

When it's hard for you to talk, you learn to choose each word with great care. If you then become a counselor, you get really good at asking short questions and making short statements that are right on point.

And there's something about a disabled counselor that disarms people. It's as though the defenses they built over time were designed for an entirely different battle, as though their fortifications face the wrong way. So, they come out of their bunkers and talk to me about themselves. Not only are they discussing a favorite topic, but they are also talking to a caring cripple, which is often thought of as a charitable act.

Many of my friends have been telling me the same thing. They tell me that they feel unseen, and sometimes, unloved. I realize that my suffering and theirs aren't that different. They feel lost and confused. They need love.

Remember, a lot of these kids have parents who are divorced. Some of them were sent to boarding school to get them out of the way of family break-ups. And some are here because no one wanted them around. It is hard to feel good about yourself when you're pretty sure your own family doesn't love you. Anyway, I think it's wrong that my friends have to feel like that. I decide to do something about it.

Every Sunday evening, the school has a ceremony called vespers, where everybody in the school community gathers at an outdoor stage in a sort of natural amphitheater. One Sunday, just after I got back from Seattle, freshly charged by another round of counseling, I ask Mr. Burr if I could lead the ceremony. He says, "Okay."

On the stage at vespers, I deliver an open invitation. I speak as slowly and clearly as I can.

"Come. Up. On. The. Stage. And. Say. What. Is. In. Your. Heart. What You've. Never. Said."

There is a pause, an uncomfortable silence, people stirring, but then, Bobby, one of my friends, walks up onto the stage. He looks around, hesitant. A lot of the guys look up to him. He's a sort of leader among the seniors. I gesture toward the audience, our classmates, our teachers. He looks down for a second before speaking. He looks up.

"There's a lot. I mean, I always sort of hid my feelings. I never really told you guys what it means to be here. Living here in this canyon with you guys. It means a lot."

He pauses, looks down at his feet again, then up.

"I've been a real jerk sometimes, I know. Sorry about that. Sometimes I didn't really think anybody cared, so I figured why should I care? Well, I do care. We all do. I know that now."

Bobby turns and walks back to his seat and there's another silence, not as long as the first, then Tom, another friend, slowly comes up. He tells us about his anxiety at having to leave his friends here when he goes away to college. Then Felicity, someone I only know a little, takes his place. And then Don, and so on, for more than an hour.

I was their guide. I had created a space where they were allowed to speak about feelings, I had opened the gate that allowed a little love and understanding into their lives. It worked.

⁓

It's graduation, and I'm the valedictorian. I could have read my speech myself but it would have taken about an hour to get all the way through it. It would have been too much to ask my friends and their parents to sit patiently for such a long time. So, my friend, Paul, read my speech for me at the ceremony.

My fellow graduates, my friends.

We hesitate to reach out and to give love to others because of the fears, doubts, and pains that we accumulate whenever we are hurt. And reaching out to give love is often not sanctioned in the social environment of today.

But we are beautiful and we need not hesitate. As beautiful human beings, we have the right to love and be loved. It solves the problem of loneliness, it dissolves fear and banishes pain. Any relationship that is not filled with overflowing love is not normal. We all have the power to reach out and make life beautiful, and we know what we need to do to achieve that end.

When we leave this place, we will miss each other a lot. We have grown very close to one another and, on this, our last day together, we fully realize it. We may not find this same closeness in the outside world.

And yet, we are very near to what we seek. We are almost there. And, as we leave this place, we take with us our wealth of human resources and our infinite capacity to love. It is within our grasp. We can be happy all the time, with all of our needs fulfilled.

When I came back from Silver Pines Camp, a powerful protective instinct was triggered in my parents that threatened to take over the parental helm completely, like a mutiny surging up from below decks. They successfully fought back the threat. I am grateful. Boarding school was good for me.

I have learned, however, that even boarding school students aren't really that independent. But I will be. I'm not going to play "Follow the Leader." I will make my own path.

17
FANG KANG

The Adventures of a High School Graduate

Summer 1971
President Nixon lifts the ban on trade with China.
Bob Dylan sings "A Hard Rain's A-Gonna Fall" at the Concert
for Bangladesh.

~

SCHOOL'S OUT.

I'm at home in Ojai.

Now that boarding school is behind me, I sort of miss it, but my world is growing wider. Some of it is in trivial things, like exchanging babysitting services for homemade granola. Like growing my own alfalfa sprouts. I mail away for brochures from every company listed in the Whole Earth Catalog. A new friend of mine drives me around to see all the communes that have sprung up around Ojai.

My dad opens our home up to people who want to learn about counseling. My brothers, Russell and Roger, get involved, but not my mom or my sister, Kendra, who both think it's artificial. Wendy, my other sister, is building a geodesic dome for her growing family up north, in the redwoods.

My dad, Roger, and I attend week-long counseling retreats that feature talks, classes, and discussions about how society shapes people's attitudes. Most of the people are disenchanted with society today. At one of the meetings, a woman waits for the right moment and asks, "What about women?" The conversation explodes into a discussion of oppression of all kinds. People talk about race, class, sex, poverty, and even disability. I am beginning to see how disability fits into the larger social puzzle. You can see more when your nose isn't touching the mirror.

~

Lots of American kids travel to Europe when they graduate from high school. Some of the guys from my class are there now, backpacking. I hear about what they're doing in Spain, in Greece. It sounds like a great adventure.

An old roommate of mine, Keo Sananikone, returned home to Laos after he graduated in 1969. He has invited me to visit him there.

I'm not so sure I want to accept his invitation, because the war in Vietnam has just spilled over the border into Laos. Most of the fighting that's going on right now is on the east side of the country, pretty far from Vientiane, the capital, where Keo's family lives. But I don't know.

~

I land in Hong Kong and catch a small plane to Vientiane. I am traveling alone.

Keo looks different than he did back at school. He has a shaved head and wears a saffron-colored robe. He's taking courses in a Buddhist monastery, so I won't be seeing much of him during the day this first week. Other than that, he's just as I remember him, a thoughtful guy with big plans.

I'm staying in a compound with his relatives and a small army of servants, including chauffeurs and gardeners.

We go to the public market. There are great piles of exotic fruits and oddly shaped vegetables, most of them completely new to me. It's crowded, lots of elderly people. Different kinds of rice, spices, coconuts, and a special kind of banana. Men are chewing betel nut, staining their gums and tongues a bright red. With all the sights, sounds, and smells, it's like sensory overload.

On a day trip outside the city, I am introduced to a Laotian doctor who runs a clinic in the jungle. He tells me that if I stay with him for two weeks, he could cure me. I look into his eyes. I try to tell if he believes what he just said. Maybe. Probably not.

Last night, I went to the movies with Keo. It was a packed house and stifling hot. Some of the people were smoking. Like a malodorous steam bath. At first, I regretted that we'd come. I thought maybe I was in for something like *The Incredible Shrinking Man*, dubbed in Cantonese with Laotian subtitles. I was bracing myself for a couple of miserable hours, but then the movie started, and I forgot where I was.

It was a Hong Kong martial arts movie, in Chinese, with English subtitles. The hero is a peasant boy named Fang Kang who becomes the student of a master swordsman. He gets really good at it, but then the spoiled daughter of the master cuts his arm off. The master doesn't know about it. A peasant girl rescues Fang, nurses him back to health, and gives him an ancient manuscript that reveals the secrets of sword fighting using only one arm. Fang masters the techniques, slays the villains, saves the master, and marries the peasant girl. Then he puts away his sword and becomes a farmer. It was called *The One-Armed Swordsman*.

I really enjoyed it.

We wandered over to the night market to get something to eat. After the theater, the night air was refreshing. The light smoke from the charcoal fires and roasting meats made the whole place seem like a giant Asian backyard barbeque. In the noisy bustle of the semi-darkness, I felt anonymous, almost invisible, and hungry. We ordered *mok* from one of the food stalls. It's sort of like a tamale, but instead of a corn husk, they use a banana leaf.

As we ate, Keo told me that *The One-Armed Swordsman* was the first movie made in Hong Kong ever to make a million dollars at the box office. I said it reminded me of *Shane*, or Clint Eastwood in *A Fistful of Dollars*. The hero standing alone against all the bad guys. But unlike those guys, Fang Kang had to beat all the bad guys with only one arm. He told me that the star, Jimmy Wang, had starred in two sequels, both of them big hits.

Chewing my *mok*, I thought about Christopher Pike, the character on *Star Trek*. The guy in the wheelchair box with the little blinking light. They don't make a lot of films with heroes like that.

And then, a thought. If I can travel alone across the ocean to visit the night market in Vientiane, I should be able to handle college okay.

18

So, What's Your Major?

Acclimating to College Life

September 1971

The Kennedy Center for the Performing Arts opens.

David Bowie's *Hunky Dory* will be released soon. *Ch-ch-ch-changes …*

I'm back in Ojai, packing my stuff to go to college.

During my last year of high school, I was already thinking about going to a college where I could strengthen my wings. In the end, I decided on Fairhaven, an alternative college in Bellingham, Washington, where I can design my own academic program and live in a dorm right over the classrooms. I can go to class by elevator. No need for a golf cart. Or a wheelchair.

I'm going to do this without a wheelchair. I'm going to walk. Yes, my right leg still isn't very cooperative, and my torso is still twisted, but I can get from here to there, if it's not too far and the way isn't too rough. I'm going to make this work.

When I walk, I feel like I'm in a potato sack race. My gait is also a bit like the traditional three-legged race, where two people run together as a

"

team with two of their legs tied together. One each. So it's like a three-legged potato sack race.

Often, to cover a short distance quickly, I resort to hopping on my left leg, which is a real showstopper. Most people have never seen someone who regularly utilizes hopping as his go-to mode of ambulation. I know I haven't. I mean, no one else hops. I try to make an art or sport of it. Usually, If I'm being watched, I tone it down. But sometimes, when someone first notices me, I may freeze in place, like a deer in the headlights. The look I get is, "Were you just…?" My response is to mime denial. "Who me? Hopping? No, no, I don't think so. No."

It rains a lot in Bellingham, and the terrain is more rugged than in Ojai. I need boots. My dad found a guy who customizes shoes. He fashioned me a pair of regular laced hiking boots fitted out with zippers. I can get them on and off by myself. It is huge for me to be able to do that. Wings on my heels. No more Apollo, Hermes now. And I got a pair of old-time locomotive engineer overalls, the striped ones. Easy to get on and off. It's colder in Bellingham, too. I'm ready for this.

Another reason I chose Fairhaven is that Bellingham is a good distance from Ojai, but fairly close to counseling in Seattle. It's like striking out on my own, crossing the frontier. Going home for the weekends won't be so easy and I will have to become more self-reliant.

I'm 17, and I'm going to leave my invisibility cloak at home.

This is it. My first morning in college.

Twenty miles south of Canada, Fairhaven College looks like an array of condominiums at an alpine ski resort. The dozen or so small dorms are surrounded by a forest of Douglas fir and are built in a ring around a commons paved with red brick. Standing here on those bricks, I half expect to hear yodeling. The cafeteria, theater, and offices are in the big building at the north end of the ring. It's a just-so-sized college of 400 students, all free to study whatever they want.

~

I don't think I've mentioned that when I eat, I don't close my mouth. I know that some people think that I am being ill-mannered when I eat like that, but I'm not. In order for me to be ill-mannered, one of two things would have to be true. Either I would have to be unaware of the etiquette concerning the display of food as it is being chewed, which I'm not, or I would have to be aware of that rule and be deliberately breaking it, which I'm not. The truth is, I can't eat with my mouth closed. I am simply eating the only way that I can.

Some people think that, because I can't eat with my mouth closed, I should not eat in public, where I run the risk of offending others. I understand this point of view and sympathize with it. I certainly have no wish to offend anyone.

Given that I must eat to survive, however, and given that the preparation of food is even more difficult for me than the eating of it, I eat my meals in the cafeteria at Fairhaven, and any fellow diners who do not wish to watch me eat shall not be compelled to watch me eat.

It seems to me that I can either eat or hide. And since I left my invisibility cloak in Ojai, I choose to eat, and let the half-chewed carrots fall where they may. And if people stare, I shall assume that they like what they see, and I shall chew on, mouth full and wide.

~

Seriously, though, starting this morning, with this first meal, I'll be eating all my meals in a cafeteria. It is an act of sheer will for me to eat in public with total strangers. It is like lowering myself into a tub full of ice-cold water. It's not easy.

I will be forced to be visible, to be seen in public, walking, eating. And not just a candied apple on a day trip to a medieval costume party, not just a single Laotian burrito at the night market, but meal after meal, day after day. For months on end. Torture.

And not only will I be visible, but I will be dependent on others as well. Right off the bat, I need help with my tray. I can load it okay. I can push it along the ledge and wrestle with the serving utensils, spilling as little as possible. But picture this. Carrying a tray with plates of food and glasses of juice from the serving line to a table? No way.

In my mind's eye, I can see this ending up like a scene in a Jerry Lewis movie, the kind where he makes fun of disability. Food everywhere. People slipping and sliding on mashed potatoes and gravy. And bussing my tray back to the trolley? Forget it. Bussing trays and hopping don't mix.

Standing here with my tray, at this, my first Fairhaven breakfast, I need help, and I am ashamed that I need help. One of the cafeteria workers notices me and starts toward me. I brace myself. Battle stations. He looks unnaturally healthy and is sporting a red bow tie. The smile above the tie looks genuine. His eyes are smiling, too. That's a good sign.

"Need some help?" Not pushy. He waits for my response. A good start.

"Yeah." I gesture toward my tray, giving permission. "Thanks."

He carries my tray across the hall and into the cafeteria, then turns and asks,

"Where'd you like to sit?"

It's early, and there are lots of empty tables. The tables by the windows that overlook the commons are the farthest from the doors. It would be nice to enjoy the view during breakfast. I glance at the table closest to the door. Mmmmm. From the back of my mind, I hear the opening bars of "Land of

Hope and Glory" being played softly on a spinet piano badly in need of a tuning. I point my left little finger to a table by the window.

"Over. There."

He carries my tray to the table, sets it down, and says, "You can just leave your tray here when you're done. Anything else you need?"

"No. Thank you," I say, nodding to emphasize my sincerity. It is always good to get permission to do that which you have already decided to do.

He chirps, "Okay," then nods and turns to leave, still smiling and still radiating that disquieting vitality.

As I sit and noisily chomp on my granola and honey, I am trying to adjust not only my expectations, but the expectations of the six other early birds in this hall with me, to the reality that at least one of us won't be conforming to the rules of table etiquette this morning. And then it occurs to me that these students are here, at least in part, because they don't want to conform to the usual rules. That's the whole idea of this college. This thought doesn't erase my lingering feelings of fear and shame. But it takes the edge off.

Fairhaven is next door to the campus of Western Washington State College. It has majors and minors, prerequisites, and academic credits and whatnot. I'm allowed to take classes there, too, but for me, it is very far away down a wet gravel trail that winds through some woods and across a field. And since I don't plan to be a nuclear physicist, and don't have my chariot with me, I plan to mostly hang out here at the ski lodge.

My educational plan while I am living here at Fairhaven College is quite straightforward.

I will study how to live at Fairhaven College.

This will be my major.

After a few weeks at Fairhaven, I ask myself: what, exactly, is so bad about people looking at me? Maybe I should just let them.

It's not that bad once you've actually lowered yourself into the tub. It's not that cold. In fact. A guy could actually get used to it. He might even like it and he might like having people look at him.

19
HOME ON WHEELS

Without Courses or Credit

Late 1971

Ashley Montagu's book, *The Elephant Man: A Study in Human Dignity*, is published.

MY ROOMMATE IS studying to be an orchestra conductor. His grandparents fled Russia in 1918 because they were Romanovs, relatives of the czar. If they had stayed, they probably would have been shot by the Bolsheviks. Then he wouldn't be studying anything.

Several of the professors at Fairhaven and a few at Western are familiar with co-counseling and some of them use its methods. I find it reassuring that they're around. I hitchhike over to Western to meet with one of them, Arthur Solomon. He looks like Mephisto and throws apples at me. I think it's due to his counseling training that he doesn't pity me at all. I return the favor.

I don't know how to register for classes and don't worry too much about it. Instead, I meet people. Talk to them. And I drop in on classes. If they're interesting, I stay. If not, I leave. No one ever questions my freedom to go wherever I want. Maybe they're trying to be nice, or helpful. Or maybe they're uncomfortable questioning the freedom of movement of a guy who walks and talks funny. No one ever checks the class list to see if I'm on it. Not even once. Maybe it's because I'm the first disabled student here and they don't know what to do. I don't have any idea, but as I see it, it works to my advantage. I go wherever I want, a free spirit, mysteriously appearing and disappearing at will. I call myself the Caped Crusader. I imagine that I have the Keys to the Campus.

I take one course about fasting and help out with a project to feed leftovers from the cafeteria to some pigs. I do not try to ride these pigs. This is a lesson I have learned.

I go north to Vancouver to try out acupuncture. It isn't legal in the U.S. It gives me a warmish glow all over, but doesn't really help. An article that I write about the experience wins an award.

I send a telex to my high school, encouraging the students there to protest the testing of nuclear weapons under Amchitka Island in Alaska. It wouldn't have occurred to me to do something like that before college. I realize now how sheltered I was, living in Shangri-La.

In the next dorm over, there's a bearded guy who wears a headband, smokes a lot, and talks endlessly about politics and philosophy. He is irreverent and tough-minded. His air of fearlessness makes me feel confident. I ask him if I can join his club. He says, "Why not." His name is Eric. We play Risk in a group with four others. He and I conquer the world together. If we hadn't formed an alliance, I would have conquered the world alone.

We hitchhike from Bellingham to Ojai.

The first night out, we end up sleeping in the bushes next to an on-ramp of Interstate 5. My dream of traveling beyond the fence like Steinbeck is realized, although in my dream it wasn't quite this cold and wet. In the morning, as we stand at the top of the south-bound freeway entrance, gray skies above, cars and trucks speeding by below, we realize that this on-ramp was almost certainly built for two farmers, neither of whom has any business in town today. We end up walking down the ramp to the freeway. After all, that is where the cars are.

A police car pulls over in front of us, on the shoulder. We go up to the window. A large policeman tells us it is not legal to hitchhike on the freeway. Eric explains about the two farmers.

The policeman studies us. Mostly me. I do my best to stand straight and still. I am swaying slightly. Eric is a little nervous. So am I. We do our best not to show it. People skills.

The policeman offers us a ride to the next, much busier, on-ramp. We accept the offer and get in the back seat. Only when he closes the door do we notice that there are no handles on the inside. Just like in the movies.

As we ease onto the road, the policeman eyes us in the rear-view mirror, then asks, "Where are you guys headed?"

Eric says, "Los Angeles, sir, to visit his folks." Meet Eric, the gracious guest.

The cop, whose stubble suggests the end of the night shift, looks out at the highway, gives his head a small shake, and says, "You fellas are a long way from home." He glances at me once more, then looks straight ahead and narrows his eyes. Then he adds, "Be careful about the rides you accept. There's bad people out there." He is squinting now.

Eric says, "Okay," a fraction of a second before I do. I glance over at Eric. His hair looks like seaweed held in place by a blue headband. As the cop turns on the signal to exit, he looks at us again in the mirror and grunts.

We pull up to the stop sign at the top of the off-ramp, then pull over onto the shoulder at the top of the on-ramp. When the door pops open, I wrestle myself out, and Eric says, "Thank you, officer," as he gets out after me with our backpacks.

Through the opened door, the cop gives a friendly, if serious look, and says, "Stay up here. Don't walk down the ramp." As the door swings closed, he gives a sort of resigned smile, another small shake of his head, and adds, "You fellas take care now," then drives down the ramp and merges effortlessly onto the damp interstate.

Policemen are generally uncomfortable around me. Many of them are afraid. The ones who swagger seem to fear me the most. In any case, they end up being like putty in my hands.

We stick out our thumbs and, in no time, get a ride with a construction guy on his way to Portland.

The second night out, we stay at my sister Kendra's place in Menlo Park. In the morning, a guy who sells tablets of benzedrine for a living gives us our first ride. He calls them "beans." He offers us some. Free. Not for us, thanks. As we zoom south on Highway 101, he talks like a fresh deck of cards being shuffled.

The third night, we end up at a Denny's in Ventura, at the foot of the mountains below Ojai. It's three in the morning. We call my parents and my dad comes to get us. And so, after a thousand miles of hitchhiking, we're there. Like there's nothing to it. Boom.

A few days later, Eric hitches back to Bellingham. I fly back the following week. As my parents and I say our goodbyes at the departure gate, they hug me and fight back tears. In Bellingham, I am alone and unprotected. They know that it's not easy for me. I know that it's hard for them, too.

⁓

Now I'm in my second year at Fairhaven, and there's a new guy on campus who has what seems to be cerebral palsy. Sometimes I see him in the cafeteria.

Sometimes in the library. I avoid him. It's like with that kid at St. Barnabas, the one with the football helmet. What is he to me? Are we members of the same club or something? It sure doesn't feel like it.

I'm used to eating in the cafeteria now. Eating with my friends is relaxing. We talk about things like Jackie Kennedy Onassis and Nixon's trip to China. We also talk about chocolate cake and the colorful characters on campus, including the guy who identifies himself only as Mogombo. He serves as a living reminder of the infinite number of ways human consciousness can unfold. He is a very different kind of different than me. But there are similarities, particularly in how he is seen and treated by society.

"Can I get you some more milk, Neil?"

"Yes. And. Cake."

There are still times when I have to eat with strangers in public. Then, I can't relax. I keep asking myself, "What do they think? Am I too strange? Do I belong here? Will they phone the hospital? What if they phone the police?" And so on. Oh, I can do it, all right, I can eat in public. But it still isn't much fun.

At a counseling workshop, I was in a skit. I played Igor, a mad scientist, complete with the dragging foot and humped back. My lab assistant was Arthur Solomon, the professor from Bellingham. He helped me discover a new world of humor and irony, the other side of my "horror."

We wanted to do it. It was funny. People laughed. And maybe it even made some of them feel better. But there's a cost to that kind of humor, the kind that seems to make fun of disability. There's something in the sound of the laughter. It shouldn't be like that. I don't think I'll do that again.

It's spring break now and I'm spending a week with a friend in Santa Cruz. I came down from Bellingham yesterday by Greyhound. This morning I decided to walk from her house to get some ice cream. About three blocks. No big deal.

But just now, on this walk, it felt like my homecoming from Camp Silver Pines. I could still walk, sort of, but every step was too hard. I'd tell my legs what to do, but they had their own travel plans, even the left one. Just keeping my balance was hard enough, never mind eating an ice cream cone.

For a long time, I have held onto the thought that, if I really try, I should be able to change my body with my mind. Despite the official medical diagnosis, it still seems incomprehensible to me that my body is not under my control. It does not help matters that "disability" is not my word. It's more like a fictitious place name in a guidebook or a misleading road sign put up by some teen-age prankster. I can't really make sense of it.

I made it back to my friend's, but now I'm completely exhausted. This is one of those times when I just have to accept reality. The reality is that I'm going to be using a wheelchair until further notice.

I spend the evening of the ice cream trek thinking about using a wheelchair. You don't realize how much time you spend thinking about the future until you suddenly have to plan for a future that includes a wheelchair. I start creating various scenarios, playing them over and over in the theater of my mind. I freeze a shot of a middle-aged me setting off for work in the morning in his wheelchair and then try to figure out the next scene, the showing-up-for-work scene. I obsessively imagine all the possible wheelchair tomorrows. The idea of using a wheelchair has taken over my brain.

On the trip back to Bellingham, I decide that I'm going to leave Fairhaven. I'm tired, and I really don't want to have to go around campus in a wheelchair. It would feel like I was going backwards, becoming more dependent. I would need more "special assistance," too, and that would feel like I was showing weakness. And it's not even clear that Fairhaven would have the kind of help that I would need, or would let me have it even if they did. I mean, I'd be the first.

I'm going to go home to Ojai. To rest.

As I was leaving Fairhaven, they told me that, because I had not registered for any of the classes I had taken during my two years there, I had not accumulated any official class credit hours. This prompted the thought that they might have broached the subject earlier, when I was roaming freely around the campus, but I said nothing. After all, I learned a lot at Fairhaven College, whether they give me any credit for it or not.

I decided to fly from Bellingham to Santa Barbara. For the first time, I was going to do it all myself. Book the flight, buy the ticket, check the baggage. The whole thing, without any help from family or friends.

When I got in line to board the plane, a United Airlines manager stopped me and took me to a small room where he expressed concern that I was traveling alone. I politely suggested that he just let me get on the plane, which was scheduled to pull away from the gate in about fifteen minutes. But he really wanted to telephone my parents to find out what they thought he should do. I tried to explain to him that I was 18 years old, even showed him my ID, but he wouldn't budge. So I gave him a slip of paper with phone numbers on it that I kept for actual emergencies. He called my parents' number. No one answered. Then he tried to call my sister Kendra. Her line was busy. So he had the AT&T people interrupt Kendra's phone call.

That's right, they broke into her call, saying it was an emergency.

I've learned that having to wait for something is not the same as being patient. In truth, I'm not patient at all.

I watched as the United Airlines manager asked Kendra what he should do. I could hear her answer.

"This is not an emergency. Just let him get on the plane."

I said, "That's. What. I. Said."

"You're sure?" The United Airlines guy asked her, pointlessly.

Kendra said, "Yes, I'm sure," at the same time that I was saying, "Yeah."

As I made my unavoidably theatrical entrance onto the crowded plane, my fellow passengers, all of them already seated and with nothing better to do, turned their heads in unison to watch me board. I imagined them bursting into song, all at once.

"How shall we extol thee, who are born of thee?"

The song got stuck in my head. I couldn't get it out. As the pilot revved the jet engines for take-off, from within the harmonic overtones of the deafening whine, I distinctly heard a choir of children's voices singing.

"Wider still and wider, shall thy bounds be set."

Flying south, looking out at the frozen tops of volcanoes, I thought about Fairhaven College, and how it had given me the education that I needed.

And as I listened to the turbofan version of "Land of Hope and Glory," the idea of a wheelchair was making itself at home in my brain, nesting in my consciousness like an alien parasite.

20

Big Break Summer

Assessing Options and Gathering Resources

Summer 1973
Congress passes the Education of the Handicapped Act.
The Weather Underground will bomb ITT's New York
headquarters next month.

~

I'm back in Ojai, living at home with my parents. Reading, watching TV, writing some human-interest stories for the *Ojai Valley News.*

My dad and I visited St. Joseph's, a convalescent home on the east end of the valley. It's set back from the road, hidden by an orange grove. I'd passed it hundreds of times, a low stone wall with a black, wrought-iron gate shaded by palms. As we wound up the oak-lined drive to a cluster of low stucco buildings, it felt as though we were entering an enchanted world.

We were met at reception by Brother Elias, who was wearing a black cassock, sort of like a long bathrobe. No collar. He had read my human-interest stories and called to invite me to visit a resident with dystonia. As we went down the hallway, Brother Elias told us that most of the residents

97

were very old and couldn't care for themselves. I'd been in a few convalescent homes, and this one seemed better than those. It was fresh and clean and the staff members we passed in the halls seemed to be good, caring people.

My dad and I met Terry Mahoney, a charter member of the dystonia club. He could barely move. My dad had told me that many people with dystonia are Ashkenazi Jews, so I rolled up right next to his bed and asked, "Are. You. Jewish?"

My dad chuckled beside me and softly said, "No, Neil. 'Ma-Ho-Ney.'"

Terry Mahoney was sputtering, unable to form words, apparently upset by my question.

I realized my *faux pas* in a belated flash. Terry Mahoney, Brother Elias, St. Joseph, Roman Catholic. My question was a reflection of my sheltered childhood. But I still didn't get why he was so upset.

Our visit with Terry wasn't long. Back in the corridor, Brother Elias explained that his order, the Brothers of St. John of God, has been helping people in need of care for more than 500 years. They are called Hospitallers.

He took us to meet another resident, a Franciscan priest named Kevin Bray, who was almost killed in a car wreck about seven years ago and has a really hard time talking and getting around now. It takes him as much energy to walk across a room as most people use to run a quarter mile. He's about half the age of the other residents. He told me it took him a couple of years to get used to the idea that he was no longer considered normal. He joked about the "youth in Asia." I didn't get it. Later, my mom explained to me that it was a joke about euthanasia, mercy killing. He said his faith is really strong now.

Brother Elias had started a group for the residents called the "Hand-icapables." They went on field trips and participated in community events and activities. I went with them a couple of times and wrote an article about Father Kevin and the group for the *Ojai Valley News*.

The most important thing that I learned from my visit to St. Joseph's and my trips with the Handicapables is that I do not want to live at St. Joseph's.

I think I'll try something else.

~

I've met a lot of people who work in the film industry, many of them through my folks' weekly poker games. Lots of other film people live around Ojai, too. Writers, actors, directors. Some of the connections go way back, like my dad's old friend who won the Oscar. When my mom was growing up in New York, her best friend was a child star in *Our Gang*. Roger knows lots of film people, too. And Bobby Carradine, a classmate of mine in high school, was just in *The Cowboys* with John Wayne and now he's working on a movie with Martin Scorsese. All of these connections make the industry seem accessible to me, like they're a natural part of life.

One of our neighbors taught acting to Jack Nicholson, who recently starred in *Five Easy Pieces*. There's a scene in it where Nicholson's character visits his father, who just had a stroke and can no longer talk or walk. He's in a wheelchair. It's a very moving scene. That was the first time I ever saw a wheelchair in a movie.

Last month, I got to play a bit part in *The Other Side of the Mountain*, a movie about a champion skier, Jill Kinmont, who, just as her career was peaking, broke her neck in a fall. She became a quadriplegic, paralyzed from the neck down. It's a true story. I'm the guy in the wheelchair in the recovery ward.

The man who wrote the screenplay is Dave Seltzer. He and I clicked. At first, our communication was slow and laced with misunderstanding. Then one day he said that my thoughts might be better articulated through a typewriter. So he got two typewriters and set them up on a street corner in Ojai. We sat side by side, so we could easily read each other's thoughts.

After a few short exchanges, Dave raised his hands from the keys, sat back, and gave me a quizzical look, one eyebrow raised. I encouraged him with a gesture toward the keys.

We typed.

> DAVE: I've always wondered how you do it.
> NEIL: How I do what?
> DAVE: You know, how you deal with it.
> NEIL: Deal with what?

He paused, glanced over at me skeptically, and must have caught the twitch at the corner of my mouth.

> DAVE: Let's face it, Neil. You are not exactly normal.

I set my smile free.

> NEIL: And yet, for me, I am exactly normal!

We went to see *The Exorcist* together. In the lobby on the way out, he told me that he's going to write a script like that, like *The Exorcist*.

It was very cool being in a movie, even if I didn't get a speaking part. Maybe next time. And there could be a next time. Maybe. Why not?

In the movie, after it became clear that Jill Kinmont was quadriplegic, one of her friends encouraged her to go back to school. I watched them shoot the scene. He convinced her not to give up. He gave her the courage to go on.

~

An article in the local paper says that community colleges in California are now providing support services for students with disabilities, including transport to and from the campuses. It says that one of them is in Moorpark, not too far from Ojai. It sounds like what was once unusual is becoming commonplace: disabled students on campus. I wouldn't have to fly solo.

The next thing you know, I'm in a van on my way to visit Moorpark College. The driver, Moses, has hair like Harpo Marx and he sings to his passengers throughout the two-hour drive. Mostly Stevie Wonder songs.

The classroom I'm visiting is on the second story. No elevator, not even a ramp. So what else is new? Moses helps me up the stairs. Late to class. Everyone is watching. Sneaking glances. Some staring. We sit in the back. It's Psych 101. The teacher asks everyone to introduce themselves. He starts in front. I'll be last. The class is antsy about the spastic in back. Finally, my turn. In a loud, confident baritone, syllable by syllable, I speak.

"I. Am. Neil. And. I. Love. People!"

In a flash, the tension is gone. Everyone smiles, relaxes.

In the words of James Brown, the Godfather of Soul, I feel good.

I've had a year off. I'm rested. It would be very easy to stay on in Ojai. Too easy.

I'm 19, and I'm going back to college.

21

OVER THE FENCE

A New College and a Road Trip

Fall 1974

Richard Nixon resigned last month.

Next month, George Foreman will meet Muhammad Ali in Kinshasa.

I LIVE IN SIMI VALLEY, two valleys over from Ojai.

I'm a student at Moorpark College, sharing an apartment near the campus with the singing van driver, Moses, and Knebel, a veteran who plays his drums like Ginger Baker.

Unlike my other schools, Moorpark has a whole community of disabled students. There's even a Director of Disabled Students, a one-eyed beauty named Zaboski. Two of my new friends are Mark Lee, who helps drive everyone around, and Don King, who is the Assistant to Handicapped Services.

Don has cerebral palsy and wears a camel hair sport coat and regular black dress shoes. He worked on Gary Hart's campaign. We arrange a dinner party in Ojai with our parents. A friend of my mom's from New

York is there as well. She's writing a book called *The Westing Game* and at the dinner asks if I would mind if she based one of its characters on me. I say, "Of course not."

In this small community of disabled people, I stand out. Most of the others have been overprotected. Remember how I said that my parents had put down the protective instinct mutiny when I got back from camp, when they let me go to boarding school? Well, some parents just let the mutineers take the helm and head for the nearest safe harbor. It occurs to me that if you decide to wait out a disability storm, you might be waiting for the rest of your life.

⌒

Eric and his girlfriend, Nora, drive down from Washington State over Christmas. We borrow my dad's camper and head to Arizona to visit Eric's parents in Sedona. We hit the road.

Our first stop is Hollywood at night, a neon watering hole in a dark desert. The sidewalks are crowded with people of every sort, dressed however they want, all of them seeming to do their best to stand out from the crowd. Wild hair, tall boots, pink leather, cowboy hats, feather boas, weird glasses, skin-tight miniskirts. Whatever it takes to be just as different as they can be. But look at me! I win the gold medal in this little Olympic competition! And I don't even have to try! It's been handed to me on a platter! Mr. Original!

I'm in the field beyond the fence. There is no day or night. There is just endless opportunity. We go to the premiere of Mel Brooks' *Young Frankenstein*. The marquee dazzles the night sky. As Gene Hackman lights Peter Boyle's thumb, we howl. When he ladles soup into Boyle's lap, we cry. Laughing at monsters, at things that go bump in the night. After the show, we cross the street and browse at Frederick's of Hollywood. Very interesting. I have never felt so free.

I've shaken the feeling of being an inmate.

~

On the way to Sedona, we stop at a Denny's in Blythe. I'm still hungry after my bowl of cereal and notice the people leaving the next table have left several sausages on their plates. Well, isn't that nice. I hop over to their table, scoop up three sausages, and return to home base without incident. Mission accomplished. It feels like breaking chains. The Denny's people didn't notice. Or chose not to notice. It was performance art, your honor.

In Sedona, we go to a guy who heals people by rearranging their spiritual energy with his hands. He rubs me and passes his hands over my body, mumbling to himself. Then he shakes his hands. He says he's shaking the excess spiritual energy off. He's doing his best, I guess, but it doesn't work. In fact, he hurt my neck. Maybe he shook off too much of my spiritual energy. I think this guy should go start a clinic in Laos. Deep in the jungle.

~

On the way back, we pull into Las Vegas after sundown on New Year's Eve and park the camper two blocks down the strip from Caesars Palace. There are no empty parking spaces any closer. We agree that we'll gamble, and that each of us will stop when we lose ten bucks.

It's cold. We're wearing parkas, stocking hats, and boots. We've been on the road for days, so we're a little scruffy. In addition, Eric still has a beard, long hair, and his signature headband. The doormen at Caesars Palace give us the stink eye as we approach, looking at my wheelchair with misguided suspicion. They clearly would like to deny us entrance, but their protocols must include some kind of override clause for spastics in wheelchairs. One wonders how often people feign dystonia in order to gain access to Caesars Palace. We breeze past.

Everyone's all dressed up. New Year's Eve parties, a live show starring Don Rickles. Women in fancy dresses, lots of jewelry, and stiff swirly hair. A lot of the men in tuxedos. The look the doormen gave us takes on new meaning. These are not our people. Where's the roulette table?

I pull up to the roulette table in the center of the betting board, right where you can bet on either red or black. Pick the right color, double your money. That's all you need to know. Forget about green. Chips are a dollar each. I have ten. Place your bets.

I put a chip on red. The little ball falls in a red slot. My heart speeds up.

I make my bet larger. Then larger. I bet ten dollars, then twenty. Over the next hour or two, I make lots of bets and here's the thing. I win more often than I lose. Really. My heart is racing now. My hands are sweaty. I have a stack of at least two hundred chips. It keeps growing.

Eric says we should take a break. We go to a nearby table and Nora, who has lost her ten dollars, suggests that I quit while I'm ahead. She points out that with the money I'd won so far, we could have dinner in a restaurant, take in a show, and stay in a warm hotel room.

Eric says, "It's your money, Neil. You won it. What do you want to do?"

"I. Can. Make. Millions."

Back at the roulette table. I can't lose. Not possible. I'm drunk on dopamine. My right leg is stuck out straight under the table. I am the master of the universe. Plugged into the cosmos. My heart is pounding now, sweat is running down my face.

"Place your bets," says the croupier.

A half-hour later, all my chips are gone.

Eric gives me his ten dollars. Within minutes, all gone.

We go back to the camper and eat peanut butter sandwiches for dinner. Then, in my sleeping bag, I reflect on the experience. It's cold. I realize that I like taking risks. I love adventure. It is exciting. My heart is still racing. I can't sleep. Now it's actually snowing outside. Only a little, but still, this is Las Vegas. I shuffle through my mental filing cabinet and find the faded manila folder labeled, "Pigs, Riding." No more roulette for me.

～

We drop by my apartment on the way home to Ojai. We park the camper next to a police car with its hood open. A cop has his head stuck under the hood. Eric walks over and the policeman tells him the starter is grinding. Eric offers to give him a jump. My dad always carries jumper cables.

The cop looks at Eric, glances over at me, pauses, then says, "No, thanks, it'll probably start in a minute. It just needs a rest."

Eric says, "Okay. But if you're here when we get back, let's give it a jump."

The cop chuckles, shrugs, and says, "Okay."

We go into my apartment, but Moses and Knebel aren't there. We drink some apple juice, pick up a few things. When we head back out, it's getting dark and the police car is gone.

We head for Ojai, Eric driving, Nora in the middle, me at the window. We're on a four-lane arterial heading toward Ventura, in the fast lane. Eric needs to get over into the slow lane to catch a right turn toward Ojai. He can't see the road behind us very well because the camper blocks the back window. He looks in the mirror outside my window, but can't tell if there's a blind spot. He asks me if it's clear.

I look and start to answer "yes," but then a car appears, so I start to say "no," but then the car zooms past. Then there's another car, so I say, "Wait." Eric tells me to lean back. This isn't a good time for slow communication. He can see the car coming up in the slow lane clearly now, its headlights are on.

Eric slows down the camper a little so the car can go past. The car slows down, too.

Eric slows down some more. So does the car.

Eric slows down to a crawl. The car does the same.

Eric says, "This is ridiculous." He looks behind him in his mirror and says, "There's no one behind me."

So he stops the camper. Right there. In the fast lane. This is a no-no.

The car in the slow lane stops, too, and immediately explodes into a display of flashing red lights. Uh-oh.

As Eric pulls the camper in front of the flashing red lights and crosses over onto the shoulder of the road, he mutters an unbelievably obscene string of graphic expletives. Then he parks the camper, turns it off, gets out, and walks over to the police car, which just pulled over right in front of us. I can see him as he walks up to the policeman's window. I can't see the policeman, but Eric looks very serious. They talk for a minute, then Eric comes back, climbs into the driver's seat.

Nora asks, "What did he say?"

Eric keeps his eyes on the police car and his face expressionless as he answers.

"He said, 'Sorry. I didn't know it was you.'"

As the police car pulls back onto the road, we all start laughing.

Eric says, "I felt like Nelson Rockefeller." And starts the camper.

It's too perfect. We are still laughing as we head back to Ojai. Eric was treated like our billionaire Vice President, who has never even seen a traffic ticket in his charmed life, and never will. And why the kid-glove treatment?

I think I know.

22

THE FLOODGATES ARE OPENING

Creativity, Identity, Freedom

1975

Saturday Night Live **debuts.**

~

I'M 21 YEARS OLD, and I'm a man.

My disabled friends at Moorpark look at me in wonder. The years of struggling against fear and shame have paid off. I'm afraid of very little now. I'm certainly not afraid of being stared at or of having someone else feel awkward when I'm around. Those problems are squarely on their side of the court now. And even though there are times when I'm a little self-conscious, what was once an open wound is more like an old war injury that only flares up when the weather's about to change.

When I was little, my full-time job was to hide, now it's to free myself.

I'm outgoing. I tell risqué jokes. I feel free to approach anyone. I start conversations with students I don't know. As far as I'm concerned, counseling gets a lot of the credit for my confidence. My Quaaludes prescription may have something to do with it, too. My friends, especially my disabled friends are surprised, sometimes shocked at my boldness. I say, "Why not? What are you afraid of?"

We have hot tub parties. And Moses often drives us to a Mexican restaurant. A big table covered with giant plates of steaming enchiladas, chili rellenos, and carne asada burritos. I am surrounded by friends, many of them disabled. I smile, and eat, my mouth wide, and smacking with pride.

We go to the movies. I go on a double date to see *Jaws* at a drive-in. I have to admit that I lost track of how many swimmers were eaten. We were very busy in the back seat. I don't think I missed much.

I take classes, too. Real classes. I am registered and get credit for them.

I took an art class. At first, I turned my typewriter into an easel, using the letters like Seurat's dots of paint. This technique gave me complete control of each point, both in the choice of the symbol and its position on the page. Very precise. Robo-pointillism, so to speak.

Then I picked up a felt pen and drew funny little pictures of faces. Different expressions. Sad. Happy. Introspective. Quizzical. I drew Harvey. Caricatures, really. Compared to the typewriter, a pen gives me less control, but more freedom, more possibility for real expression. I realized as I was drawing that, in one sense, I was just making marks on paper. I realized that the art of drawing is really just making marks on paper. Even if the marks are made by Leonardo da Vinci, they are still essentially marks on a piece of paper. Maybe that sounds obvious, but I'd never thought of it like that before.

Then I had a revelation.

These marks that I make on paper are art. My art. And this drawing is worthy to be called art, worthy to be in books, worthy to be hung in a gallery. Because this art, this funny little picture of Harvey, is a direct expression of my thoughts, no one else's. It came from this mind, and was expressed through this hand, which, of course, has a mind of its own.

So. My art is unique. No one else can draw like this. And the art of drawing, all of the graphic arts, really, are not thought of as being linked to disability at all. But when I create this art, I automatically make that connection. This is a bold thought. And funny, too.

I decide that not only will I write, I will draw.

In a film class I was thrilled by *Seven Samurai*, the story of a village that hires a band of samurai to fight marauding bandits.

Another course centered on Bronowski's *Ascent of Man*. In a powerful moment, he put his hand into the mud of Auschwitz and "touched" the remains of millions of long-dead victims of the Holocaust. Never before had I been so moved by a TV show.

A Day in the Life of Bonnie Consolo was shown on Disability Awareness Day. It blew me away. She's like Aphrodite. No, Venus de Milo. She is a living goddess without arms. The rock-opera *Tommy* made me feel included. *"See me. Feel me. Touch me."* I am on the outside, too, and I do feel strange. This deaf, dumb, and blind kid is like a one-armed swordsman.

I start writing a column for the school paper and, at Harvey's urging, I began putting out a newsletter about counseling and disability. At first, I called it *Handicapped, Not Incapable*, but, after a few issues, changed it to *Complete Elegance*. I try to replace the negative expectations that society has for disabled people with a more positive view, one that unlocks potential.

～

There's a slope on campus. Not high, but steep. There's a long, paved walkway that traverses the slope. I use it all the time to get to class. Today, however, I've decided to go cross-country.

I wheel myself over to the middle of the top of the slope. People start heading my way, so, right then, I go over the edge. I ease myself down the slope slowly, very carefully. It is steeper than I thought. Not to worry though, one of the many silver linings of dystonia is that all that clenching and flexing turns your muscles into steel cables. I'm strong. I let the wheel turn a little more, get a little farther down the slope, then stop for a breather. By now, people are at the top saying, "Stop him! Don't let him go! He'll kill himself!"

A guy in a UCLA sweatshirt working his way down the slope toward me is shouting, "What are you doing?"

"I'm. Being. Very. Careful," I say calmly.

"You can't do this!" he pleads.

"Actually. I. Can," I say, in my most reassuring tone.

"You're crazy!" he concludes in frustration.

"Don't. Worry. I'm. Not," I reply. I am the very model of a man who's rational.

"Why don't you go on the walkway?" Now he looks like a father whose daughter is about to go out on her first date with a letterman in full rut. "It's safer!"

"Because. I. Don't. Want. To," I answer, batting my eyelashes, relishing the role of the teenybopper debutante.

We go back and forth for a while. It's like improv theater. Except he's not acting.

"Come on, man!" He's almost whining.

Finally, I say, "Okay. I'll. Let. You. Carry. The. Chair. Down. And. Yes. I'll. Walk."

Boy, is he happy now. He'll remember this for the rest of his life. I look around and see all this honest emotion that is so rarely expressed. I'm grinning inside and I'm honored, too.

Dystonia is more than just a word. It's how you feel when you have it. It's how the world treats you and how you treat the world when you're not able to speak easily or move easily. One old medical dictionary defines dystonia as "sustained involuntary muscle contractions of antagonistic muscle groups, leading to grotesque posturing or jerky, twisting, and intermittent spasms," but it's not really that, it's so much more. Besides, this use of the word "grotesque" makes me laugh.

∼

It's spring, and this is so cool, and so weird. I'm at a weekend conference about disabilities in education at a four-star hotel in Los Angeles. All expenses paid. Professionals are here to talk with one another and learn about the latest in the field. I was invited to attend. This is all new to me. This isn't a dorm or a campus. This is the "real world."

I read that Albert Einstein once asked, "What does a fish know about the water in which he swims all his life?" Good question. I think that I've learned a little something about water. In a way, I've lived both in it and out of it. So maybe it's not so strange that I was invited. I guess I do know a little something about the latest in the field.

I go alone to a restaurant to eat. This, all by itself, is unusual. You almost never see a person with a disability in a restaurant. Not with a disability like mine, anyway. I sit at a table, order a cheeseburger with fries and a vanilla milkshake. I am served. So far, so good. Then, I notice that I have the fries, but no ketchup. And not a waiter in sight.

So.

I stand up.

I hop over to the wait station.

I get the ketchup.

I hop back.

I sit down.

And start eating. Like there's nothing to it.

I notice that there's this guy watching me. His hair is blow-dried; his glasses, wire-rimmed. Corduroy sports jacket. No tie. He gets up, comes over, and introduces himself. Ron. He says he's the Coordinator of Disabled Student Services at Solano Community College. We talk for hours. And then, what's this?

He offers me a job as a counselor at his college. Just like that.

I guess he was very impressed with my version of the old "get the ketchup" job-interview trick.

Imagine that. Me. An official member of the American workforce.

I take the job. I start in the fall.

~

It's supposed to be International Women's Day, but at Moorpark we decide to call it Bicentennial Human Day. The ceremony is on a stage in front of hundreds of people, many of them disabled. Ms. Zaboski asks me to speak.

I hesitate, not sure why she asked me. Everyone's watching me, expectant. I'm not sure what to say. Pins drop. Then I think about the way disabled people are portrayed in movies and on TV. As shy, lonely victims, hiding in the shadows. As weak and childlike beings without thoughts worth hearing. And, suddenly, it comes to me. I know what to do. I guess Ms. Zaboski chose me for a reason.

I rise out of my chair, muscles flexed, of course. My strength is reflected in my stance, in my visage. My right arm is tight against my chest, the wrist bent double. My left arm is freer, moving in arcs at my side. Now I am standing, mostly on my left leg. Every muscle is taut. In my lowest, strongest voice, I speak.

I talk slow.

"Moses. Watched. Me. Take. A. Photo. He. Said. The. Art. Wasn't. The. Photo. It. Was. Me. Taking. It. We. Are. Becoming. More. Visible."

Some of them get it. Some of them don't. I stand, I move. On display.

"I. Am. Not. Shy." Driving home the point.

A couple of people say, "Yeah!"

"Fear. Keeps. People. Down." I say this loud.

From an uncertain silence, a lone voice. "Right on."

"We. Aren't. Hiding. We. Are. Getting. Stronger." I emphasize the last word.

"Yes!" Several voices now.

Then I raise both arms and stand with my legs apart. Rising. I sway a little, then steady myself. "Change. Is. Here!"

Now they're standing. Clapping.

"*Yes!*"

"We. Are. Emerging!" No one is in the shadows now.

The crowd cheers. I am now part of a movement. They are shouting. These are my people.

23
DROID POWER
Working for Change at the Grassroots Level

Fall 1976
Steve Jobs starts selling Apples.
The Concorde takes off.

I'M LIVING IN A RENTAL in the Suisun Valley, just up the road from Solano Community College.

I'm working at the college. I'm 22, and it's my first official job.

My roommate is my boss, Ron, the guy who hired me. Usually, he makes us sack lunches, and I cook dinner. Tonight's special? Garbanzo loaf with red sauce and tofu cabbage soup. I am now a gourmet vegetarian chef. Or at least a vegetarian chef. I seem to enjoy eating garbanzo beans as much as I enjoy saying "garbanzo beans."

Our rental is in Mankas, California, a country crossroads with a small store on one corner and a seasonal fruit stand across from it. All the rest is orchards, mostly almond. The store also doubles as a sort of deli that sells shepherd's pie as an entrée. The store's owner is our landlord. He used to rent this place to a Mexican family who worked in the small peach orchard outside our back window but found out that he could get more from a couple of gringos who work at the new college.

The rental is really almost a shack. Single-wall construction. The board that you see on the outside of the house is the same board that you see on the inside of the house. It's just the other side of the board.

At night, it's really quiet. No cars, no neighbors. I love our little shack out here in the sticks.

❧

On my first day, I hitchhike to work. It's only two miles. I roll out to the Mankas Corner Store and stick out my thumb. Within minutes, a car pulls over, the driver puts my portable chair in the trunk as I get into the passenger seat, and we're off. He drops me off at the curb right in front of the college. Oh, yeah. It was a police car.

Usually, Ron and I ride together to work. As part of my contract, the college gives me my first electric wheelchair. Very cool. The college has a lift van that I can ride home in.

Ron and I share an office. Officially, my title is Teaching Aide, but Ron didn't hire me to do his busy work. You could say that I'm Ron's right-hand man. But just as I exercise little control over my right hand, Ron exercises little control over me. Let's just say that Ron has a spastic right hand. Or maybe a semi-autonomous right-hand man is a better way to put it. He hired me to do things that he can't.

My primary job is to change things around here. Radically. To change the way the college accommodates the physical and developmental differences of its students. To change the way the faculty thinks about those differences. To change the way students think about those differences and think about themselves. Everything that I do, from the smallest task to the biggest project, is focused on these changes.

With the encouragement of Dennis Banks, who's teaching up the road at UC Davis, I organize a Student Union, like a lounge, so that people who otherwise might feel like outsiders, isolated and alone, have a place that is theirs, where they can be part of a community. Sometimes they come to it as a temporary refuge from the wider community, where things can get a little rough. Where self-doubt and self-loathing can sound persuasive. Dennis helped found the American Indian Movement. A few years ago, he helped organize the occupation of Alcatraz.

I write for and edit *The Rising Tide*, a newsletter Ron urged me to start. It's supposed to be for disabled students, but its real target is much wider, raising issues of race, class, gender, and sexuality. Of humanity. Everything in it is intended to move the reader toward the goal: A world in which the differences between people are not seen as justifications for exclusion or oppression, but as expressions of the richness of humanity and opportunities for growth and celebration. It also runs announcements for the Chess Club and classified ads. "For Sale: inflatable bathtub. Only $275. Portable. Does not leak."

I organize a faculty workshop, an in-service. I try to root out pity, to allay fears. Changing the minds of those who tacitly dismiss the whole program as a thinly disguised charity is a priority. I demonstrate ways that they can foster respect, strength, and independence in their students.

We role play. I model smashing preconceptions about the abilities of their students. It isn't always what I say that matters. Sometimes, my presence alone compels people to look at themselves and others in a way that otherwise would not have been possible.

I also learn that, properly placed, a single word can be the fulcrum that upends the way a person sees the world. I am spending more time lately waiting for just the right moment to say just the right word. As a man of few words, I must choose mine carefully. And I learn about the power of metaphor. More broadly, I begin to see the need for art to help build our pride.

I start a peer-counseling program, using techniques I learned from Harvey to help the community here become happier, stronger.

Although I was not raised in the Jewish faith, I was told by a counseling group leader that I am, nonetheless, a Jew. She said, "Your dad is Jewish. Your mom is Jewish. You are Jewish. That's all there is to it." This new part of my identity makes stories about oppression more real to me, and somehow more personal.

Still, being disabled trumps being Jewish.

We go on lots of field trips. Lots of socializing. We go to restaurants. We are putting our bodies and souls into the wider society. Even when I am not working, I am working.

I go to see *Marathon Man*. Laurence Olivier plays a Nazi war criminal who tortures a Jewish graduate student, played by Dustin Hoffman. The Nazi wants to know if his safety deposit box full of diamonds is being watched by government agents. As he drills into the student's unanesthetized teeth, he asks, "Is it safe?" Over and over. I am repelled by this scene. And drawn to it. It is not easy to admit it, even to myself, but I enjoy movies with scenes like this.

We go to see *The Omen*, David Seltzer's answer to *The Exorcist*. We also see *Pumping Iron*, *Saturday Night Fever*, and *Star Wars*.

The *Star Wars* bar scene is a revelation. Sentient life forms from all over the universe relaxing together. Talking, laughing, drinking, squabbling. Their common denominator isn't how they look or talk, it is consciousness itself. Exactly.

When Luke and Obi-Wan are accosted at the bar by a misanthropic extra-terrestrial simply because they are human, I am amazed. Then the bartender demands that the droids leave because, "We don't serve their kind here." Androids become the wretched of the galaxy. "Sentient Life Forms Only. No Droids Allowed." Spielberg is showing us the way.

I know it was meant to be funny, and it was, in a way, but I actually felt a flash of anger at the way R2-D2 and C-3P0 were bounced out of that bar.

Injustice does not seem that funny to me.

24

THE WORK FORCE AT WORK

I Learn about the Limits of the Law

Spring 1978

Ben and Jerry open their first shop in Burlington, Vermont.

***The Westing Game* will be published this summer.**

❧

I'M AT THE KITCHEN table in Mankas.

I just had an eye-opening adventure.

I took the bus to the Department of Rehabilitation office in Fairfield. I was curious.

After watching a fluorescent light in the waiting room flicker for twenty minutes, I was directed to a windowless office where a man dressed entirely in polyester sat behind a desk made of gray metal. He looked up from a piece of paper and the corners of his mouth turned up slightly. He looked very earnest. I was slightly alarmed at how earnest he looked, but I don't think I let it show.

He told me his name was Mel. He asked me how much money I had in the bank and how much money I got each month. The numbers were small, teaching aides don't make much. I said that I worked at Solano College. Then he asked me about my medical history and my disability. I was frank and concise in my responses. It's called dystonia. Yes, my condition is more or less stable. No, there's no known treatment. This is it, I indicated, what you see right here.

He paused. Looked at me for a moment. Up and down. Then he looked me in the eye. I could see a glow in his eyes, like a nightlight in a hallway.

Then he said, "I'm really sorry, Mr. Marcus, but your case is too severe for our department to be of any real assistance to you. Our purpose here is to help people so that they can eventually get into the workforce. In your case, that just isn't a realistic goal."

Dipping into my oceanic reservoir of patience, I explained again to Mel that I was already working. I even showed him my job description. It didn't work.

Mel had jumped to the conclusion that I was employed in a sheltered workshop and no amount of evidence was going to coax him to jump back. He could not stretch his mind sufficiently to get it all the way around the idea that the 24-year-old man seated in the electric wheelchair right in front of him, whose limbs were off on self-chosen missions, who had just taken about a minute to give an all-but-incomprehensible seven-word answer, possessed skills so valuable that an institution of higher learning would give him a paycheck to secure his services.

Cutting me off mid-syllable, he told me again that he was very sorry, but his department had nothing to offer me. He looked at me very earnestly and said, "My advice to you is to stay right where you are. It is the best that you will get."

On the bus, on the way back, I thought about my conversation with Mel, replaying it over and over in my mind. I found it incredible. I thought about his job, his role, his mindset, and what I could do to help him see things differently. I began drafting a letter to Mel.

I'm sitting at the kitchen table in Mankas, writing the letter. I'm going to send it to Mel. And I'm going to send a copy to his boss. And a copy to the governor. I decide not to suggest that the Department of Rehabilitation open a branch office in a jungle in Laos, but a bureaucracy is no better than its most inept bureaucrat.

The phone rings. It's a friend from work named Chuck. He says we should skip work tomorrow because it's St. Patrick's Day. He wants to go bar hopping together in San Francisco.

I say, "I'm in."

❧

We take a Greyhound bus from Solano to the city, my portable chair stowed below in luggage. Crossing the Bay Bridge, I look over at Chuck. He looks like a mountain man who has come to civilization for a short visit. At six-four, and well over 200 pounds, he is an honest-to-god titan. Formidable. He is also blind.

Chuck tells me that he has always been a true ally of the underdog. His soul, he says, is absolutely intolerant of injustice and callousness. He tells me that when he lived in Washington State, if someone in a bar said something that he found offensive or insulting, he would trash the place, just tear it apart. I look carefully at Chuck, asking myself if this story is true. Maybe. Maybe not. But, you know, there's something about the set of his jaw.

Emerging from the diesel fumes of the bus station, I tell Chuck there's an Irish pub across the street. Chuck says, "You're a good scout, Neil!"

I watch the traffic and monitor the crosswalk lights. "Now!" We cross the street. He helps me with the six-inch curb.

We go into the bar and Chuck orders two draft beers. The burly owner of the bar says we can have one beer each, but then we have to leave. He says that it is nothing personal, that he isn't prejudiced, and that his wife is in a wheelchair, too, but that he, nonetheless, has to ask us to quietly leave after we finish our two beers.

I blink. I can't believe what I just heard. That I don't drink never even enters into it. The bartender is smiling as he says all of this, but it is the smile you seen when a Doberman Pinscher sizes up the UPS man. He adds that he "really doesn't want any trouble in here."

Over the course of this presentation, Chuck's face has gone from white to pink. By the time the bar owner is finished speaking, Chuck's face is the red that you see on a Nebraskan farmer's back after his first day at the lake following a long winter. Sensing trouble, I intervene, quickly convincing Chuck that it's best for us to go. He reluctantly agrees. Something tells me that he's only agreeing because he's not yet drunk.

We go into another bar a few blocks away and Chuck again orders two draft beers, this time adding, "Make them boilermakers!" This means that each beer comes with a shot of whiskey that Chuck drops into the beer, shot glass and all. No trouble from the bartender here. He's more of an Italian greyhound than a Doberman.

After two boilermakers, Chuck tilts his head, smiles, then starts chuckling, shaking his head. "Well, well, well," he says softly, smiling broadly. "You know what we got here, Neil? We got ourselves a gay bar." The curls of his hair are bouncing in amusement. Sipping my orange juice, I look around, and realize that he's right. The decor, the outfits, the pairings. I can't help feeling that I should have worked it out first.

Then I sense that I am being watched. There's nothing new in this. People watch me all the time. Usually, when they see me notice them watching, they quickly look away. So I decide to watch the watcher, so to speak. I look, and at a table over Chuck's shoulder, sure enough, there she is, a thin woman with short hair and great beauty, seated alone, staring at me. Our eyes meet, they lock, and she doesn't look away.

A bit taken aback, I look over at Chuck and say, "There's. A. Woman. Behind. You. Staring. At. Me."

With no hesitation, Chuck says, "Good scouting, Neil. Let's go over and introduce ourselves."

I orient Chuck to the target table and we go over. Her name is Alex and she invites us to join her. The accent may be from New Jersey. Her short dark hair is in a Peter Pan cut, meticulously unkempt. Her dark eyes have just enough shadow, liner, and mascara to suitably frame them. Her nose is fine and straight. Chuck launches into a surprisingly convincing imitation of an experienced, but sensitive, man-of-the-world who has joined the crusade against sexism. Alex responds semi-automatically to Chuck's conversational gambits, never taking her eyes off me. When Chuck pauses to sample his fourth boilermaker, Alex leans toward me with a small smile and whispers, "You have the most wonderful eyes. They are sooo deep."

Chuck asks me which way to the men's room. I hold out my arm and he feels the direction I'm pointing it. "The left door," I advise him.

"Got it," says Chuck, "I'll be right back." He rises from his chair, swaying slightly, then makes his way toward the restroom. It's like he's tacking into the wind. I watch, making sure he veers to the port. He does.

Alex moves her chair closer to mine and asks me about myself, starting with where I live, what I do. She puts her hand on my arm. Her nails are very short, with glossy red polish to match her lips. She is really interested in me. "Fairfield," takes about a half a minute to be transmitted and the same again to be received. Mankas and Solano are too obscure. Then I have to decide. Teacher? Counselor? Teaching Aide? I go with the easiest to say, and to make myself understood. "Teacher." Then Chuck comes back and discovers that while he was gone somebody has stolen his cane.

"What kind of world is this, anyway?" Chuck wants to know, once again red-faced, this time, glistening with sweat. On his feet. "I mean, come on! Steal a cane from a blind man?" He seems more angry than disappointed. Then he has another question. "How messed up is that?" Except he didn't say "messed." I resist the urge to shout "Right on!" It would be a mistake at this juncture to egg him on. I think he is about to blow.

The moment Chuck's soliloquy began, the bartender had launched a one-man search party to recover the missing cane, and now, just as Chuck was about to show us the unimaginable degree to which things could, in fact, be messed up, the barkeep speaks. "Sir? Here it is. Here's your cane. It was in your backpack."

Such a revelation might have humbled a lesser man. Not Chuck. He simply holds out his hand, accepts the cane, barks, "Thanks," and takes his seat, saying, "Ah, yes, Alex."

I butt in to tell Chuck that there is another blind man sitting at a table not far from us, nursing a beer, wearing shades and a battered cowboy hat. Chuck is immediately interested. The bartender tells me the guy's name is Blind Bernie. I tell Chuck, so Chuck greets Blind Bernie and introduces himself.

"Hi, Bernie, I'm Chuck. Sometimes they call me 'Blind Chuck.'" Blind Bernie doesn't say anything. Doesn't even move.

"Hey, Bernie? My name's Chuck. How you doing, man?" No response. Just facing the wall.

"Hey, man, what's your problem? What, you're too good to talk to other people?" Nothing. Not a twitch. I sense that, deep within Chuck, magma is once again accumulating. The bartender is on his way back now, with the inner ends of his eyebrows drawn together and crawling upward, the very essence of empathetic fear.

Alex says, "He just doesn't want to talk, Chuck, okay? Leave him alone, for Christ's sake." Lines of annoyance appear in the thick make-up around her eyes and mouth.

Chuck is full throated once more. "For the love of God! All I did was say 'hi' to him. What the heck is wrong with everybody?" Except he didn't say 'heck.'

The bartender has arrived. I think he's actually a bartender/dancer. It's in the way he moves. On the balls of his feet. Almost on his toes.

In a firm, steady, terrified voice, he tells Chuck that he's very sorry, but if he doesn't calm himself down right now he's going to have to call the police and he doesn't want to do that, but he will, because the other customers shouldn't have to put up with all this yelling and shouting, and if he can't control himself, he's just going to have to leave right now, because enough is enough, and that's enough, and he's going to have to call the police.

Chuck draws himself up to his full height, looks down toward the bartender, inhales deeply, pauses. Then he goes full mountain-man.

"What has happened to us? What has happened to our humanity? Where has it gone? I'll tell you what it is! It's city life! Cold, unfeeling city life! Where nobody knows anybody! Where everybody's a stranger! Where human connections are broken! Where human connections are never even made! Where nobody talks to anybody except to buy or sell something! Or to buy or sell someone! Or even to sell themselves! Nobody even touches anybody unless it's been paid for! Where everything's made out of metal and cement and plastic, and smells like garbage and toxic chemicals and untreated raw fear! Come on, Neil, let's get out of here! This place stinks!"

With that, Chuck turns and walks into my chair.

As soon as we step off the bus back in Fairfield, a car pulls in behind us. The driver pops his trunk and pulls out a portable wheelchair. Weird. Wait a minute. That looks like mine. What the heck? The driver wheels it over to us with a bashful smile on his face.

"I saw it fall out of the luggage compartment about ten miles back," he says. "I pulled over and got it. It's a little banged up, but it still seems to work okay."

I'll always remember this St. Patrick's Day as the first and only time that I ever called in sick to go bar hopping. And the only time I got thrown out of a bar like R2-D2.

❀

I am in our shack in Mankas, looking at my monthly paycheck. I am thinking about work.

The more highly others value the product of your work, the more money you get paid for it. That's not a hard and fast rule, but it's a rule. Brain surgeons are paid more than barbers. And, like it or not, people connect the amount of money that a person gets paid with the value of that person. And if this check is any indication, I'm not worth much. Not nothing, but not much.

Underlying this is the expectation that workers must function perfectly. The subtle law that we all live by, knowingly or not, is that we have to perform our work very efficiently. Let's be honest, if you think about it, this means it is expected that we will not be disabled.

The result is that those of us who do not function perfectly feel bad. We have failed to live up to the expectation. We are breaking the subtle law. We are, as these things are measured, outlaws, and are, quite literally, worth less. To make matters worse, people who are not disabled look at us and feel bad, too. Not only that, they feel scared. Disability frightens them. Like it's catching. And they project these fears and bad feelings back to us, the disabled, which only makes us feel worse.

And the message goes around and around. Disability is bad. Echoing. Amplifying.

Bad, bad, bad.

Sitting here at the kitchen table in this shack in Mankas, I see it so clearly. It is an enormous negative feedback loop that all of humanity is trapped in. If only that first expectation could be erased, that first law repealed, the bad feelings will stop and everyone, whether disabled or not, can live happier lives. It's clear to me. It's wrong that so many people feel this way. I've got to do something about it. I'm not sure what, but it has to be something big.

❧

My new friend Barney comes to visit during the summer break. He is a fellow dystonic. We understand each other in a way that no one else can. All of the things that we have both been asked to explain a thousand times and have never been able to communicate satisfactorily are already known. They are our shared reality. Talking with him is like drinking a tall glass of cold water after a long hike in the desert.

We go canoeing on Grizzly Bay, in the estuary of the Sacramento River. We have to work very hard to keep the wind from sending us to the south shore. Paddles going this way and that. We briefly consider entering the Paralympics in the tandem canoe sprint event, then think better of it and laugh.

Barney tells me about the 504 Sit-in at the Federal Building in San Francisco last year. Led by Judy Heumann, 150 disabled people occupied the Department of Health, Education, and Welfare offices. Barney was one of them.

He tells me how the occupiers had to help each other. Preparing food. Helping each other eat. Administering medications. Preventing bedsores. Cleaning things up. When the pay phones in the offices stopped working, people used sign language out of the fourth-story windows to colleagues in the plaza below to get out press releases. To kill time, there were wheelchair races in the hallways. After 28 days, the longest sit-in in U.S. history, the government agreed to implement Section 504 of the Rehabilitation Act of 1973. Barney rolled out of the building with the others. Victory.

We are rising.

∼

It is the fall of 1978. I move out on my own and rent an apartment near the college. Ron is great, but I've depended on his help for everything. It is really challenging for me to live without help. Shopping, cooking, cleaning. Washing dishes. These everyday tasks are not easy for me to do. I must do them all very slowly and very carefully.

I go outside my apartment to the sidewalk, and a bunch of stray kids pass by. They notice me and stop. Then they sort of adopt me, and take me along with them. They're living on the edge, and I realize that I am too. It makes me realize how vulnerable I am.

I set up a little security system in case I get stuck. I told Ron that when I'm in a jam and need help, I'll call him and say, "I'm in a phone booth." That is our code for, "I need help." Now, I probably *will* be in a phone booth when I say it, but I may not be.

The reason I chose this phrase is not that it tells him where I am, but that it is an easy phrase for me to say because the *m*, *n*, *f*, and *b* have similar lip positions. In an emergency, I'll probably be nervous, and it will probably be hard for me to talk, so I need the code to be something that I can say even if I'm all stressed out. Therefore, when I say, "I'm in a phone booth,"

I've instructed Ron to ask me, "Are you in a phone booth?" and not to be surprised if the answer that I give is "No."

We even rehearsed it:

> NEIL: I'm in a phone booth.
> RON: Are you in a phone booth?
> NEIL: No.

I'm a little uncomfortable living alone. I mean, I can do it. But it is really hard, and I think that, maybe, I need a change.

～

I'm in my office, working. A woman steps through the door. She is short and thin, with delicate, almost elvish, features. We talk for a while. Her name is Gayla. I can tell that she needs to talk, that she has things that she needs to say to someone. I listen.

She starts coming by my office every day during lunch. She talks about her life, her feelings. I listen. Sometimes, she will cry, sobbing uncontrollably, then, all of a sudden, explode in laughter. More and more, she hands me cryptic notes about her marriage, her everyday life, and about love. They are like disjointed poems, with parts missing.

She often pulls at my unbending right arm as though it were hers, as though it was meant to be free, not clamped against my chest. As though if she could just free it, then she could be free, too.

She joins my counseling network. I become her counselor. When we walk together, she shuffles her feet on the pebbles. I meet her husband, and her two children, Aidan and Rianna.

I am 24. I have never had what I think of as a "real" girlfriend. To me, whatever this is, whether it is love or something else, it is intoxicating.

Gayla and I go to see the movie version of *The Wiz*. In the darkness of the theater, I am not transported to Oz. What I see are African Americans taking control of their own cultural images. As I watch Michael Jackson's scarecrow dance up the stairs, as I watch Diana Ross sing, I realize that I am watching Black culture being created by Black artists. As I listen to Lena Horne sing, "Believe in Yourself," I can think of no reason that disabled artists shouldn't be able to build their own culture. And use it to break the giant negative feedback loop.

Below my review of *The Wiz* in *The Rising Tide*, I add the following invitation:

> Wanted: Your opinion as to whether the Scarecrow, the Tin Woodsman, and the Cowardly Lion in *The Wizard of Oz* should be put in the category of "handicapped." Anxious for a debate on the pros and cons of this subject. Marcus, Neil, 169 library.

I would have liked to hear Diana Ross sing "Over the Rainbow."

~

It is clear that Gayla and I are both looking for a change.

25
CHANGING THE TIMES
Learning the Ropes

Summer 1979

McDonald's sells its first Happy Meal.

This fall, Iranian students will take over the U.S. Embassy in Tehran.

~

OUT OF NOWHERE, I got an offer to study computer programming in Berkeley. The offer even included a small stipend to help with living expenses. So I moved into a ground-floor apartment in Berkeley.

With Gayla.

And Aidan and Rianna.

I am confused about my feelings for Gayla. Is this love? I don't know. I'm 25 now, almost 26. You would think that would be old enough to know, but I guess it doesn't work that way.

When she cries on my shoulder, I find it hard to separate her need for me from my feelings for her. Sometimes I think I love her, sometimes I'm sure I do. But then I wonder if I would have these same feelings for her if she didn't seem to need me. It's wild. Part of what's going on is that there's a certain disability chic now. Some people think it's cool to be associated with disabled people when they're not. Sometimes I think Gayla is taking pride in being in a relationship with a spastic man. That would make me a sort of fashion accessory.

❧

Berkeley sits on the eastern shore of the San Francisco Bay, looking into the sunset behind the Golden Gate Bridge. Berkeley. What a great place to make a change. Where to start?

How about the moment in 1964 when Mario Savio jumped on top of a police car to address the crowd of students blocking it? Student activism was born that day.

The following year, when the first U.S. ground troops were sent to Vietnam, hundreds of students marched. That was the start of the anti-war movement.

A few years later, some 10,000 demonstrators closed down the building where army draftees reported for duty. In the end, the draft was stopped.

In 1969, thousands of women marched up Shattuck Avenue to celebrate International Women's Day.

Later that year, the Third World Liberation Front organized a student strike, demanding an academic program that addressed the needs of minority students.

A couple of months later, the counterculture and the establishment squared off over the fate of the People's Park. It continues to be an unofficial park.

In 1970, after the Kent State killings, classes at Berkeley were canceled for six weeks as anti-war rallies swirled through the campus.

Berkeley's a good place to make a change.

Take Ed Roberts.

Ed got polio when he was 14, in 1953. He was paralyzed from the neck down except for two fingers and some toes. He still uses an iron lung, a big metal cylinder. He can be out of it for hours at a time, and use a wheelchair, but needs to sleep and rest in it.

When he was in high school, he took most of his classes by telephone. They almost didn't let him graduate because he hadn't taken PE and driver training.

After a fight with the Office of Vocational Rehabilitation, Ed was admitted to UC Berkeley in 1962. He was housed on-campus in the old infirmary. At first, he was the only one there. By 1969, there were eleven others using iron lungs in there with him. By then, Ed was working on his PhD.

They started to go around Berkeley together in their wheelchairs. They called themselves "The Rolling Quads." Sort of like an outlaw wheelchair club. They demanded curb cuts in Berkeley. What good is a sidewalk if you can't cross the street? The curbs were cut. They started the Physically Disabled Students' Program, which, within a few years, led to the creation of the first Center for Independent Living in the world. Run by and for disabled people to help us live independently. The Berkeley CIL opened its doors in 1972. Now there are CILs everywhere.

Ed Roberts is like David; the system was his Goliath. For a while, he was one of the directors at the Berkeley CIL, but now he's the head of California's Office of Vocational Rehabilitation, the same outfit that tried to lock him out of college. This means that Ed is now Mel's boss. Mel, who told me not to expect much.

Ed Roberts changed things.

~

Our apartment is near a small park, near enough that I can get there in my portable chair. The power chair had to stay at Solano. With this one, I have to go backwards, pushing with one foot while looking over my shoulder. It works, but it's pretty slow going. To go further afield, we put the chair in the back of Gayla's station wagon. I also ride the public buses. It isn't easy, getting a portable chair on and off a bus, but I can do it.

Five days a week, a van picks me up and takes me to my computer classes at the Berkeley Center for Independent Living. One of my fellow passengers is Judy Heumann, a leader of the 504 Sit-in, who calls me "Marcus." Now she's one of the directors of the CIL. At first, I'm a bit star-struck. She suggests that I write children's books.

All of my programming instructors are disabled. One teaches from his portable bed. Very cool. Lots of corporations are hiring disabled programmers for big bucks. Dell, IBM, Levi Strauss. Many others. I am seriously considering becoming a computer programmer who is an artist on the weekends.

Maybe I can make millions.

∼

Gayla writes letters to prisoners. While I see this as a humane act, I wonder if in some part of her mind, maybe a part that is hidden from her, she sees me as another prisoner she's writing to. Or maybe there's a part of her that's locked up, a part that she sees when she looks at me. I really don't know.

At least once a day, Gayla says, "Neil, you really need to grow up."

This inspires me to be more independent. I answer, "Okay, mom." We're being playful, joking around.

We joke around like that a lot.

26

SLOTHS

Problems with Communication

Early 1980
After 28 years, the soap opera *Love of Life* airs its final episode.
Superman II, starring Christopher Reeve, will come out later this year.

MODERN LIFE IN BERKELEY is fast-paced and impatient. Everyone just expects it to be like this, including me. I become impatient with myself.

As I speak, I hear the words to be spoken in my head before I speak them. I calculate the shortest way to give voice to the thought. I select the words that are the easiest words for me to say that can still convey the meaning. I select those with the vowels and consonants that are the easiest for me to say, that include them in the order that rolls most easily off my tongue. I am doing all of this so that I can be understood.

For example, if I'm talking with my friends Daniel and Todd and I want to refer to Bertrand Russell's notion that truth is a tentative working hypothesis, I don't, because Russell's name is almost impossible for me to say.

Words that start with the "B" sound are hard enough by themselves, but to follow one with a word that starts with "Ru" will end up being unintelligible. On the other hand, words that start with "S" are relatively easy, and it's easy to follow that with any word that starts with a "D," especially if the "D" syllable is followed by an "L." So instead of bringing up Bertrand Russell, I say Salvador Dali. This is easy for me to say because my unruly tongue stays at the front of my palate. I could just as easily have answered "garbanzo beans."

A peripheral effect is that conversations with me often go sailing off the rails. After my mention of Dali, Todd may say, "I think what Neil is trying to say is that Dali sublimates and disassociates logic. Right, Neil?"

In this context, "Yeah," would be the easiest thing for me to say.

Have you heard about Mayan hieroglyphs? By the time the Spanish arrived, people had forgotten how to read them. There were hundreds of these distinct, seemingly meaningless, square symbols. There didn't seem to be a pattern.

Now they've figured out that inside each square there are two or more small, stylized pictures of objects. When you blend together the initial sounds of the names of these objects in Mayan, you are actually saying the word contained in that square, sort of like a Rebus puzzle.

So, in Mayan, many things begin with the sound "Ka." The written language can use a picture of any one of these things for the syllable "Ka." And each Mayan scribe was free to choose which picture to use.

In a way, my speech is like Mayan hieroglyphs, in that any given word is rarely spoken the same way twice. Endless combinations of lung, throat, tongue, jaw, and lips are used to create the same syllable. Unlike the Mayan scribe, I rarely get to decide which little picture, which sound, comes out next.

⁓

I continue counseling in Berkeley with Charles, a professor of classical literature. He has given me some wonderful direction. We both relax completely and do everything in super slow motion, even talking. When a part of my body has a spasm, he holds that limb until it passes.

Have you ever seen a three-toed sloth in action? There's not much to see. They travel about 40 yards a day. They make Tai Chi Chuan look like time-lapse photography. Well, when Charles and I work together, we look like two three-toed sloths doing physical therapy.

Thank you, Charles. You showed me a way out.

〜

I used a new kind of telephone today. It is called a "Telecommunications Device for the Deaf," or TDD. First, I type something on the built-in keyboard. Then the AT&T operator reads what I typed to the person I'm calling. Then that person talks to me, the operator hears it, and types what is said so that I can read it on the built-in screen. We continue this way, back and forth.

I don't like the name. This device isn't only useful for deaf people. I'm not deaf and I certainly find it useful. Sometimes it's called a TTY after its predecessor, the teletype. This is a better name. The TTY is simply another way to communicate. For me, it is a tool that allows me to solve complex problems, such as making flight reservations.

I called United Airlines on their dedicated TTY number. I successfully booked a round-trip flight to Santa Barbara. The operator, the ticket agent, and I are a band of insurgents operating in the shadow of a faceless communications conglomerate. We have a sense of solidarity. I signed off with, "Have a good day! SK." "SK" is Morse Code for "over and out." Another doorway to freedom opens. Yes!

I still haven't figured out how to program a computer quickly.

27

FREEWHEELING

Getting Around

Late 1980

Ronald Reagan has won the presidential election.

John Lennon is living in the Dakota Apartments in New York City.

~

A FEW DAYS AGO, I bought a used electric wheelchair. This chair was really built for a child. Very basic, very slow. No class today, so I'm taking it out for a test flight.

I head west from downtown Berkeley, toward the Bay. I'm in the city, on my own at last. I am traveling solo, over the fence, into the fields beyond. Dealing with traffic and crosswalks. I use the curb cuts. I shop a little, buy some snacks. It is revolutionary for me to be out here.

I tip over. Don't worry. I'm not hurt. I get up. Get going again. Then the left wheel neatly slices through a mess deposited by a local dog. Oh, joy. As I'm cleaning it off, a motorized bed comes zipping down the sidewalk. I think, "What?" There's a guy flat on his back on the bed with mirrors angled in front of his eyes so he can navigate. To control the electric motor, he manipulates a joy stick with a stylus he's holding in his mouth. Quadriplegic. He stops next to me. We look at each other.

I'm thinking, "Jeez, and I think I have problems."

His look says something like, "Wow, look at this poor guy."

Each of us is wondering if the other guy can talk at all. He looks in the mirror and sees the paper towel in my hand resting on the wheel of my new chair.

"Bummer," he says, followed by something I can't understand at all. Then he makes a throaty "Aaach" sound as he almost leaves the sidewalk into the path of a passing Volvo. I try to put on my relaxed face.

The bed stops again. He says, "I'm Mark O'Brien."

I say, "I'm. Neil."

Then he says, "See you around, Neil," and he's off. Just like that. As I watch him go, I label this a "Berkeley Moment."

I travel about two miles west. This is a big deal. I am 26 years old, and I am now mobile. I have access. I am independent. I am free. This is the first of many journeys. I'm going to learn to use the buses better. Learn to use the rail system. Learn to use taxis. Learn how to get to the airport in my chair, onto an airplane and go wherever the heck I want. Using technology for mobility, access, and independence. To jump fences. This is a very big deal.

I got on a bus last week. I was in my new electric wheelchair. Even with the lift, getting on was hard. It took time.

As I was getting settled, the driver asked, "What's your stop?"

As clearly as I could, I said, "Eighth. Street. Studios."

She gave me a look that indicated my effort to make myself understood had been unsuccessful.

Fair enough, I thought. I'll give it another try. "Eighth. Street. Studios."

She got out of the driver's seat and addressed the man in the seat closest to me. "Do you know what he said?"

As I was transferring myself into the bus seat next to him, the man turned his palms upward, shrugged, pursed his lips, raised his eyebrows, shook his head slightly from side to side, and said, "No." In that order but as one fluid motion. Like there was nothing to it.

As I've said, my speech becomes less clear when I am stressed, and I was starting to feel stressed. But, I thought, here goes. Once more into the breach.

"Eighth. Street."

She looked at me. Then she rummaged through every cardboard box in her mental store-and-lock, looking for something, anything that resembled the series of sounds that I had just made. This went on for a full second before she turned and addressed the other passengers. "Does anyone here understand what this guy is saying?" In her tone I detected a pinch of exasperation.

I was in the bus seat now, strapping my chair in front of me. She was eyeing the chair and me with purposeless suspicion when a guy near the back of the bus said, "Did you say Eighth?"

I smiled and gave a quick left thumb up.

The driver slowly shook her head as she returned to her seat, and we were off.

At Eighth Street, I stood up and tried to unstrap my chair, but the strap got caught in the frame. Oh, great.

The driver said, "Next time, stay in your wheelchair. Now sit down."

I responded with a firm "Okay," then sat down in the bus seat again as she wrestled with the strap.

She got the chair free, and I got in it. As I maneuvered the chair on the lift and out the door, I gave her a very strong look. Actually, I glared at her.

Just outside the doors, I turned just in time to see her face as she said, "Don't you flirt with me!"

Her tone seemed to be an odd mix of scolding and mocking, of a shared joke and cruel fear. As she closed the doors with a pneumatic whoosh, and turned to the front, her lips formed a small and crooked half-smile. I'm not sure I want to know what the other half was.

Life is rough.

Most people are more willing than this bus driver to try to bridge the gap between my speech and their ability to understand it. I have learned that people who are confident that they can figure out what I'm saying generally do.

Some things are easier to say than others. For example, it's easy to say, "Hi, how are you?"

It's harder to say, "Eighth Street Studios."

The written rules and laws that govern our actions are important, and changing them if they're unfair is important, too. But it is more important to change the feelings of the people who wrote those unjust laws in the first place, and who support them now. If those feelings can be changed, then changing the laws is simple. Change the feelings and there will be no opposition. Then we can settle out of court.

But how do you change the way people feel?

Maybe I could have had a career as a programmer and made millions. Now, I'll never know. I dropped out of the programming course. Or flunked out. It was not my cup of tea. I'd rather be an artist than a programmer. In a way, I think I already am an artist.

After I dropped out, I got sick. Shingles. I had a bad rash of red spots. It hurt. Like my nerves were on fire. It's also contagious. I think it scared Gayla. Maybe she was worried about her kids getting it. They'd just had the measles. Anyway, she moved out. So I'm on my own again.

My dad found me a co-op apartment near the CIL, just around the corner from People's Park. My new home. In my chair, down the elevator, out the door, and I can go anywhere.

For me, it's the perfect place to get serious about becoming an artist.

My dad is hunting for a "cure" for dystonia. While he knows that there are a lot of quacks out there preying on people, he tells me that some of the non-traditional approaches look promising. He says he'll keep me posted.

He is determined to help me, and I don't think he's going to let it go.

28

TOUCH THERAPY

The Elusive Mind/Body Cure

Summer 1981

Prince Charles and Lady Diana just got married.

MTV will start broadcasting tomorrow.

~

THIS IS HAMPSHIRE College in Amherst, Massachusetts. My dad and I drove here from Ojai a month ago. We've been staying in the dorms while I get physical therapy from Moshe Feldenkrais.

Moshe combines dance, movement, and manipulation to treat the nervous system. He believes that by manipulating the body, you can change the brain itself.

Moshe has been teaching advanced classes here over the summer break. People have come from all over the world to see him. Some are parents who have brought their children, hoping that Moshe can help them where others have failed. Many of the kids have cerebral palsy. Some who came are practitioners who hope to learn from the master. The most favored students observe Moshe's sessions closely and get to hear his running commentary, what he calls "the elusive obvious."

My dad started to tell Moshe all about my diagnosis, going into detail about the symptoms, medications, and surgeries, but Moshe raised one hand and said, "Beh." He thought the medical explanations were wrong. Moshe was the intellectual equivalent of a battle tank, plowing through any obstacles that lay between him and his objective. In the end, he agreed to work with me twice a week, twice as much as anyone else.

During my sessions with Moshe, it was like he was guiding my body. I felt like he was telling me, "Do not give up. There is hope. You can move with more freedom. I will help you."

Harvey's method and Moshe's seem complementary to me. Both seek to heal damaged emotions, one through the mind, the other through the body. I think both can be effective. I loved getting to know Moshe, and wasn't really surprised or disappointed that dystonia proved to be too stubborn for his method.

I'm 27 now and not as focused on finding a cure as I once was. I've found that many people who focus their lives too narrowly on finding a cure often don't do much of anything else.

One of Moshe's star pupils is Gabriela. She sat in on my sessions. At a party in the dorms a few nights ago, we sang "The Boy from New York City" together. Afterward, she walked over to me and asked me if I wanted to stay with her for three weeks in an apartment in New York City. She told me that it was hot and muggy in New York that summer and that the apartment didn't have air conditioning. She said we'd have to go to cafes to have Italian ices to cool off.

Do I want to stay with her? God, yes. I'm chomping at the bit!

"I'll go!"

I'm sweltering in a tiny ground-floor apartment on Mott Street in Little Italy.

A small window at the back looks out on a little courtyard where two spindly trees are wedged between tall brick walls. They're leafed out, but look like they could use more sun.

The apartment is so tiny that the kitchen counter has to be shoved to one side to access the bathtub. Extension cords snake all over the place to the fans, lamps, radio, and refrigerator. Mostly fans. All day long, we listen to the banter of the DJs as they play the big hits on AM top forty radio. We sleep in the loft, like two pieces of toast. Even with the fans going all the time, there's no need for sheets, and I'm as happy as I've ever been.

Bette Davis eyes.

Instead of having sit-down meals, we forage up and down the street, stopping in shops and bakeries, buying whatever smells or looks good. The bakery next door supplies us with hot, fresh bread. From little markets we pick up cheeses from everywhere. All kinds of yoghurt and granola. And fruit. I know they don't grow it here, but nowhere has better fruit than New York. Some of these peaches were probably grown in Mankas.

We take walks. My new chair is much faster than that old kid's model. We can really move. Past pawn shops, liquor stores, sweatshops, a tannery, a pork store, nothing but pork. "Excuse me, sir, could you tell me which way Greenwich Village is?" A deli. A jewelry store. A chic boutique with mannequins sporting orange jackets with avocado trim. Like spacesuits from the 1940s. Hats, just hats. Punk fashion. Leather, distressed denim. Shoes. A cigar store. It's like everything in the world is for sale within a few blocks of us.

With the heat, people move out of the brick-oven apartment blocks and onto the stoops and sidewalks, spilling into the street. People from every-where. All ages, all sizes, all colors. Kids running, chasing one another. "Hey, lady! Your kid threw a rock at my window!" Accents, languages. Laughter.

Whistles. Cars cruise by, arms hanging out windows. Humidity. Boys leaning on cars, handling their cigarettes with choreographed nonchalance, talking to girls passing on the sidewalk. A blonde in jeans hides her smile with her hand, wary of expressing her delight. Completely alive. From nowhere, a whiff of sausage, diesel, and garlic. A thin boy walks by, swinging his hips, boom box on his shoulder. Michael Jackson has nothing on him. Four old ladies in flowered dresses sit on the stoop in aluminum lawn chairs, saying nothing as he passes, squinting in envious disapproval. Then, someone tucked away somewhere in the windowed canyon walls above cranks up Kool and the Gang. As if on cue. All the way up.

Celebrate good times, come on!

The excitement. The heat. The life. I'm still stunned. What a wild few weeks we've had together here in Little Italy. It has filled me with optimism about life, about independence and possibility.

I'm going to write more, to work more. There's a lot that needs to be done.

29
DISCO IN MY SOUL

Discovering the Art of Dance

1985

Moshe Feldenkrais died last year.

~

I'M IN BERKELEY. I've been thinking a lot about beauty. And dancing.

In the 1930s, my mother took classes from Martha Graham, who is sometimes called "The Picasso of Dance." She taught my mother that you must translate the energy of life into action that expresses who you are. You channel the life force. She said that if you block the process, the expression will never exist, never come into this world. She told her that dance expresses who you are more completely than anything else. And your job is not to compare your expression with others. Your job is to keep your expression authentically yours.

Your job is to keep the channel open.

Around 1984, I started going to dance classes and workshops at the Skylight Studio at 8th and Dwight in Berkeley. On Friday nights they held dance jams there. Open to everyone. I'd go in and join a crowd of dancers that seemed to have been hand-picked to showcase the rich and endless variety of humanity, with a spotlight on disability, just about every kind of disability you can think of. This was a very new thing for disabled folks. It was a revelation to me.

No one is hiding here. No one is using the tried-and-true techniques employed to avoid attention. No stealth tricks here. No bushes. No back row seats near the exit. Leave your invisibility cloak at the door. No disappearing acts here, folks.

Contact improvisation really takes off at these dance jams.

My girlfriend Devva, a fellow spastic whose every move is filled with grace, drives us there. Watching her on the dance floor is like watching Joe Cocker on fast forward. She is a blur of motion. We dance together on the floor. Smooth as silk, our spasms moving in rhythmic harmony. Use what you have. Make contact. Improvise. It fits us perfectly. Devva and I touch, and balance, and roll around, using each other as leverage to move in ways that are only possible together, and only for us, right now. Lots of physical contact. Moving as one, our bodies are connected with this new art form.

Contact improv. Move, touch, lean, and balance. Then move some more. No routines. If it were one way, fixed and directed, not fluid and open-ended, it wouldn't work at all. Here, no one leads. Everyone leads. Together. Otherwise, it would be like Nureyev lifting Fonteyn in Giselle, as though she is a sack of potatoes. One way action. Contact improv is back and forth, push and pull, entwining, then unwinding, alive. Just as all true dance is alive.

In 1985, I went with my friend Paul to the Anarchist Cafe on Mission Street in San Francisco. It has an "open mic," where you get 15 minutes to say or do whatever you want. I roped Paul into getting onstage with me, to interpret. Speaking very slowly, as my counselor Charles had taught me, word by word, I told the audience about the monarch butterfly.

"Birds. Don't. Eat. The. Monarch. Butterfly. They. Find. Its. Taste. Disgusting. This. Helps. It. To. Survive. Birds. Leave. It. Alone," I told them, as Paul interpreted. My gestures were expressive, expansive.

The audience was listening intently, struggling to make sense of me. "Butterfly? What's he talking about?" They were on the edges of their seats. Then, my eyes very wide, I told them about the viceroy butterfly.

"The. Viceroy. Looks. Almost. Exactly. Like. The. Monarch. So. Birds. Leave. It. Alone. Too," I said, striking exaggerated poses, some intentional, some not, bringing the anecdote to life. Very dramatic. Very kinetic. It was dance.

"But," I said, then paused, "Birds. Don't. Know. That. The. Viceroy," —a long pause— "Tastes. Good!"

A look of recognition lit up the faces of the audience. Loud applause. On the way home, I told Paul, "I. Had. Them. In. The. Palm. Of. My. Hand."

I loved being on that stage. In the spotlight. I think I was born to dance, and to perform.

I begin to dance in my chair, and out of it, and with it, wherever, whenever. And as I dance, I begin to discover that this is in my blood. My body knows how to move. It knows comfort with other bodies. I can get or give help in movement. I am comfortable with touch and with voguing poses. I live in contact improv now. It works for me!

I am a dancer!

I am keenly aware that there are people who are puzzled when I say this. They say to themselves, "A spastic dancer? Is he serious?" Well, I'm not kidding. The more I dance, the more I realize that I was meant to dance.

Who is the better dancer: Mikhail Baryshnikov or James Brown? The question assumes there is a single yardstick we can use to measure beauty. The question assumes there is a frame around art, and suggests that the bits outside the frame can be cut off and discarded. This assumption limits our ears, our eyes. It limits our perception of art and the way we experience life.

Is the expression authentic? Does it express something unique? Is it true? These are the questions. And these questions will forever challenge those who hold up their yardsticks to measure beauty and use rectangular frames to chop off the more chaotic and unconventional part of the canvas that doesn't quite "fit in."

I cannot dance like Mikhail Baryshnikov. But Mikhail Baryshnikov cannot dance like me. Nor should he try.

But I'll try anything. I'll play any part, take any role. I'll be Travolta or Baryshnikov, or even Tina Turner. I am undaunted. And that boldness, that fearlessness, that willingness to try anything may be what people see, what they are dying to see.

On the stage. Center stage. In the spotlight. On fire.

Behold! I choose not to be shackled by doubt and fear! Behold! I choose to be lifted by my dreams! I choose to allow the life force to express itself through me!

And that, all by itself, is beautiful.

I promise myself. I will develop as a dancer. I will open the channel.

I go to People's Park, to the space among the trees.

And I dance.

30
DRAWING CONCLUSIONS

Putting Disability in the Picture

1986

Andy Warhol is putting the finishing touches on a series of prints inspired by *The Last Supper*.

❧

I'M SITTING AT MY dining room table, staring at a white sheet of paper. In my left hand is a black felt marker. I'm thinking about beauty. And drawing. I'm thinking about becoming a graphic artist, a painter.

So.

A gifted young painter went to work on a large canvas. He worked on it for months, painting over complete sections again and again. When the painting was finally finished, he hid it under his bed. He would only take it out to show to his closest friends, then roll it up and stick it back. Most of them thought it was ugly.

The painter was Pablo Picasso. He finished the painting in 1907. It was not displayed until 1916. The painting, *The Young Ladies of Avignon,* is now widely considered to be the single most influential work of art of the last century.

What was once thought to be ugly is now beautiful.

What changed?

Not the painting.

We changed. People changed. The way we see changed. Another way of saying the same thing is that the culture changed, but that misses the point. The point is that we *can* change. The point is that we do.

This is very good news.

I think drawings generally have two components, a representation of something from the outer, objective world of matter and an expression of something from the inner, subjective world of consciousness. This means that every drawing is essentially autobiographical. The pen tells about the person holding it every time its tip touches the paper. So when I draw, no matter what I draw, I am drawing about disability.

It is baked in the cake.

My head is always full of ideas clamoring to get out. I am a cyclone of ideas. When an idea comes and I don't get it out fairly quickly, it often simply goes away. And more ideas keep popping into my head all the time. So I feel this sense of urgency. I have to get my ideas on paper right away, before they disappear.

You might think that if I were to draw really fast, I could get all my ideas out before they're gone. But often, if I draw fast, people can't tell what I am drawing. So I generally draw slowly. Just as I speak slowly and have to choose my words with care, I think carefully about which ideas to draw, which one to draw next, and what lines to draw. And as I draw, I try to keep in mind that if I am too self-critical, too burdened by doubt, the gates of creativity may slam shut.

My drawings are not ornate. Necessity has nudged me toward the technique used in minimalist Zen painting, the kind done with a few strokes of a sumi brush. With this technique, I too can create an image like *Nude Descending a Staircase* with a handful of bold strokes. And in my drawings, each stroke is as clearly mine as my reflection in a mirror.

What do I draw? I draw the ideas that bubble up in my brain. I don't have to go to them, they come to me. Then the images that express these ideas appear in my mind's eye at the exact moment that the ink touches the paper. These images are like words. They are symbols that express an idea. And one of these images can contain as much meaning as a book full of words.

What do I draw?

Imagine.

A neolithic painting of a hunt. The mastodon and three hunters with spears. One of the hunters is using a wheelchair.

At the back of a public bus sits a man in his wheelchair, reading *Black Like Me.*

A guy in a wheelchair atop a surfboard, tube-riding a monster wave.

A little cafe with a long ramp that wraps around it, leading to the entrance. At the foot of the ramp is a man in a wheelchair, saying, "Build it, and they will come."

I create simple drawings that help people see.

I am still sitting at the table, staring at the white sheet of paper in front of me.

Today, printed pages are mostly filled with bad images. Thoughtless images hawking deodorant. Pictures of people delighted by their toothpaste, or their insurance company.

Imagine that everything you see around you is designed to exploit and oppress humanity, to deprive people of power. Now flip it, make what is called 'disability' into what people actually want or need. Touch, for example.

The AT&T commercial suggests that we, "Reach out, reach out and touch someone." That's it. Or consider the elegant access of the inviting spiral ramp that is the Guggenheim Museum in New York City. Or a seemingly simple thing like a drinking straw, that empowers, that liberates. Or braille art, beauty at everyone's fingertips. Or the beauty of Wyeth's depiction of his neighbor, Christina, who couldn't walk. That's us, I say. Not negative. Artful. Positive.

Today, disability culture is hidden. It is under the bed.

I want it out there, out in the open. Drawing is another medium to help me fulfill my mission to push toward a vibrant disability culture, bursting with style. I want to see images of disability culture everywhere. In magazines, on TV commercials, in shop windows. I thirst to see larger-than-life, full-color images of disability culture in the ads on the sides of buses and on billboards.

I put the tip of the pen on the paper.

And draw.

31
Down All the Day

Despondency

Mid-1980s

Perestroika.

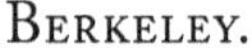

Berkeley.

Morning.

I wake up, but don't want to get up.

So don't.

I lie on the floor. I don't want to eat. I don't want to fight with my body. Arm wrestling with yourself all day, every day, can get very, very old.

So stay on the floor.

One hour.

I don't want to deal with my surroundings at all. Today, it looks like a diabolical obstacle course.

So stay here.

In a way, I'm an invisible person. You can't tell who I am or what I do or what I think. People often tell me they had a friend or relative "like me," but more likely he or she is simply invisible, too.

An hour and a half.

Staring at the changing light on the ceiling of my apartment and half-listening to the faint sounds of the neighborhood eight stories below, I feel time ooze by. The refrigerator starts to hum. I left the windows cracked overnight and can tell it will be hot again today.

Don't get up.

My fellow Americans, the state of the union is not good.

In this great land of ours, millions of people are oppressed every day simply because they are different, because they are what is called disabled.

We are the people left behind in the snow. The people who are sterilized, lest we reproduce. The people you don't look at, you pretend not to see. The people who scare your kids, who scare you. We are the people who are slaughtered, lest we taint the blood of the master race.

Two hours.

I am so tired of people projecting all their unrealized idealism onto me. Am I supposed to do it for them? I won't do it.

So don't.

People come up to me all the time and talk cheery nonsense. And I smile and nod and act all cheerful like I'm having fun and life is fun. But what does fun have to do with it? They're messing with me. With my dignity. With my manhood. My life is hard enough without having to put up with their mindless drivel. Sometimes I just don't have the patience for it.

Go cheer somebody else up.

People are curious. Even when they sense it may be impolite, they ask me questions. The most common one is probably, "Are you in pain?"

My stock answer is, "No, I'm invincible."

But the truth is there's a deep pain in a body that isn't working properly. It's a force at work telling you: Stop. This is wrong. This posture, this motion doesn't follow the rules. This is pain, as I see it. It is a force that thwarts things that don't fit in the natural order. It is a fundamental, physical truth.

The humming stops. For the time being, the refrigerator has decided to call it quits.

Don't move.

Two and a half hours.

I can't stand it anymore. I can't stand this feeling of being frozen in darkness. My doctor prescribed a mild tranquilizer for days like this.

I take one.

After a while, I thaw out a bit and carefully prepare a note for the computer store. I take the elevator to the lobby, and roll out onto the streets of Berkeley, already bathed in summer sunlight. On my way to the store, I realize that part of the reason I'm in such a funk is my new computer. I can't use it yet. It's overwhelming me. It's so powerful. I think it may be smarter than me.

Up pop all my old insecurities, like crazy hand puppets. My mind starts racing: what about this? What about that? All these details. Don't forget to do this! Don't forget to do that! A chorus of anxieties, jabbering together in falsetto. Sometimes I don't handle change very well, I guess. Jibber-jabber. And change is unavoidable.

I am the only customer at the PC store. Good. I hand my note over to the manager behind the counter. He reads "I'd like a Glidepoint mouse, please." He looks at me and, with a twinkle in his eye, turns to his four employees and says,

"All right, all hands on deck, NOW!"

He turns back and grins at me, watching for my response. I grin back. The Glidepoint will come in the mail in a week.

On the way home, I bump into my friend Daniel in his wheelchair. What a powerful spirit he is. This world seems too small for him. While I've met bigger people, none of them seem to occupy as much space. His thick black beard reaches very high on his cheeks, then, from the eyebrows up, not a hair. We talk about the new gallery that just opened near the campus. Then he says, "Let's go for a ride!"

We zoom up Telegraph Avenue in our chariots. Past cars, motorcycles, tourist buses. Past signs that tell us where we can and can't go. Past shadows, reflections, visions, and people sleeping on the street. We go wide around a group of power walkers, swinging their arms comically high. Then into the Berkeley campus, through Sather Gate. As we head down the long hill near the library, we gather momentum, really flying now, past picnickers, past lovers making out on the lawn. Some people smile and wave, like in a home movie. I'm really glad I got those wheel bearings replaced. They're really humming now. The bumps in the path feel like waves on a lake. And in this one moment, for the first time today, I feel good. *Zzzzzzzzzz.*

On my way home, I swing by Mark O'Brien's. He's been using an iron lung since he was six years old. And, more recently, a motorized bed, the one he was in when I first met him. He's a writer, too, and I'm hoping he'll review my new children's book about a princess in a wheelchair who is taught to ski by a friendly dragon. We swap a few anecdotes. He tells me to bring over a copy of the book. Cool.

Back at home I check my messages. Roger, my brother, tells me about a change in train schedules. He says he'll keep me posted. *Beep.* My girlfriend tells me she misses me and asks me to call soon. *Beep.* A voice says, "How'd you like to come home to AT&T?" *Beep.* Then Todd calls and says he's coming by. "Let's meet in the lobby," I say.

In the cool of the lobby, the conversation drifts from neurology to metaphysics and back. Then, as Todd develops the thesis that technology makes progress inevitable, Sam, a neighbor, steps out of the elevator, walks to the desk by the front door of the lobby, sits down, picks up the phone, and begins dialing.

Todd is saying, "The human mind, with the right technological support, can do anything," at the same time that Sam, talking into the telephone, is saying, "I'm having a heart attack. Please send help."

Todd stops talking, stunned. He and I look at each other. My mind races.

"Is there anything we can do?" Todd asks as he hurries over to Sam.

"No. Nothing." Sam's color is wrong. He's taking pills and rubbing his left shoulder. He puts his hand over the middle of his chest. We sit with him.

The firemen come. Then the paramedics. Tubes. Oxygen. IVs. Heart monitors. They take him away.

We are both still upset. Todd says goodbye, then leaves. I take the elevator home.

I wind up lying on the floor again, still in a state of shock about Sam's heart attack. Feeling down again. It's getting dark outside.

People often tell me that I have a lot of courage, especially when they first meet me. I have no idea what they're talking about. Me? Courage? I'm just living my life.

This morning, I felt like I could not go on. I felt paralyzing fear flowing in my veins. It was affecting my mind, my will to live. I felt lost in it. My body was freaking out, too. Frozen and erupting in spasms at the same time. Should I get up? No, it's too hard, stay on the floor. But I need to get out. No, it's better to stay in. It's easier, safer to stay in. Learn to like it.

But that's like death. What's the point of living if you're not going to do anything but lie on the floor? Love is that way, too. Should I call her? No, it's too hard. But you need love. You have to get up off the floor. You have to live. You have to love. You have to get up. You must act. You just have to.

I get up off the floor. I cook dinner and eat.

Tomorrow I'm heading over to Santa Cruz for a weekend counseling workshop with Harvey. I need this workshop. I really need to get charged up. I go to bed and call my girlfriend, who says, "Hi!"

32
Who's On First?

The Student Becomes the Teacher

Spring 1986

The Challenger disintegrated.

The nuclear reactor at Chernobyl exploded.

JUST A MONTH AGO, at the age of 32, I led my first disabled liberation workshop in Arizona.

I reminded the group that all of us want to be loved. I set it up so that people would take turns being "the center." I went first.

As "the center," I controlled everyone's actions. I told everyone to love me unabashedly. I chose the people I wanted to sit next to me. I pointed to the place on my cheek that I wanted to be kissed. I named the songs I wanted to be sung to me and chose the singers. And I basked in it all the way a cat luxuriates on a patch of sunlit carpet on a cold morning.

A few hours later, after everyone had taken a turn as "the center," I asked them all to introduce themselves to each other, and then we went outside for lunch. Right away, people started feeding each other. They were giving directions, saying what they wanted. "Now a slice of apple! No, the other one!" It was starting to look like the eating scene in *Tom Jones*. Then some of them started playing tag. Some others started spitting watermelon seeds, not as a contest, but for fun. It was as though a playfulness had been released, a sense of joy. We were all free, for now, from that subtle sense of desperation that underlies the lives of so many people in the world today.

Leading the workshop in Arizona helped me trust my own instincts. It showed me that my life has given me knowledge to pass on. It also changed my leadership style. Now, there is no set format other than helpful encouragement. Helping others find their own way. Free-form.

∽

I'm in Santa Cruz.

I'm here for a counseling workshop for teachers and leaders.

It's the last night of the leader's conference in Santa Cruz.

Harvey is about 70 now. He stands straight, head up, shoulders back. It makes him seem taller than he is, and he's not short. He's built like a boxer. No flab on Harvey. The lines on his face are from years of smiling.

He doesn't give speeches. There is no prepared text for Harvey. He talks about the role of oppression in society. When he responds to questions, his answers are laid out logically, methodically, often at some length. Step by step. By the time he's done, you get the sense that the question has been thoroughly answered.

When he talks with people, he is always focused. Oh, he laughs and jokes, but nothing distracts him from his mission. Not excuses, not tears, not even laughter. Whether he's counseling someone privately or in front of a large group, he is all about helping people regain their power, and ending oppression in all its forms. Harvey stays on point.

At the session today, I raised my hand.

"Yes, Neil?"

"How. Does. One. Get. Help. If. One. Has. Trouble. Talking?" I asked.

It took me at least 30 seconds to ask this question.

Harvey's response was to say, "Come on up." This is what he says when he is inviting you to talk about the question that you asked.

Another person might have heard my question, noticed the trouble I had asking it, and detected the ironic intent. It was a setup line.

"Come on up," was what he said. And extended a hand.

I rolled up, and then stood up next to Harvey, my abstract cubist form providing a nice counterpoint to his symmetrical realism.

"Neil. You have to utilize your great intelligence and your boundless creativity …"

He started out facing me, but turned toward the group as he warmed to his familiar theme.

And then I realized that Harvey had turned to that theme because he didn't know what to say to me. He reached for it because he was stumped.

I looked at him and, for the first time, saw all of him. I saw a human being, with the imperfection that may be our species' defining characteristic. I saw a fellow human stumbling forward into the misty unknown.

"… and focus your energy on finding solutions to overcome these obstacles to clearly communicating …"

Now, I could have nodded. I could have quietly let things run their course. Played my assigned part and then returned to the group. But something about this new view of Harvey, the mere mortal, allowed my innate theatrical sense to take over. My inner jester was set free.

So.

I turned and looked at my fellow participants, raised my eyebrows, and rolled my eyes.

"… your needs, whether those needs are physical in nature, such as the need …"

Most of them were still looking at Harvey, but a few had noticed the eyeroll, and looked a bit surprised. Their looks asked, "Is Neil making fun of something Harvey just said?"

So then.

I squinted my eyes as though mystified by Harvey's words, looked quickly at him, then back at the audience. And then I mimicked Harvey. I stood straighter. I held my head up as high as it would go and put my shoulders back as far as they would go. I raised my hands a little, so that they were about the same level as his. Then I imitated Harvey's facial expression. Eyebrows up, eyes slightly hooded, mouth and chin confident, not quite arrogant. I was an abstract caricature of Harvey. More of the group noticed. More surprise.

"… for food, or drink, or warmth, for example …"

At this point, several members of the group suppressed their laughter, a few with only partial success. Harvey noticed it and glanced over at me. I looked at him, wearing his face, and he didn't recognize it. He kept on going.

"… or emotional in nature, such as feelings …"

Still speaking, looking around now for the source of amusement, worried that he was losing control, Harvey turned again toward me just in time to catch me give a sigh, glance down, and then slowly turn my head to face him, brows arched, eyes meeting eyes.

"… of isolation or of loneliness or of alienation …"

And I became his reflection in a mirror. Like him, I gave my head a quick, barely noticeable shake, and raised my shoulders an inch, all the while wearing his face of puzzled exasperation.

And Harvey kept on talking, looking at me now, giving it his best.

"… or of being lost …"

Then Harvey stopped speaking.

We looked at each other. At each other's eyes.

The audience was watching, confused.

Harvey, this man who knows so much about people, was suddenly seeing himself in a new light.

I realize that I am a long way now from doing corny skits about Igor.

This feels like a kind of graduation ceremony.

I think I may be ready to try out my theatrical skills on the real thing.

When I mimicked Harvey today, I thought I was highlighting the issue of disability. As performance art, it worked, in a way, but I was using him as my unwilling straight man. I got a little carried away. He taught me about power and I used it against him. I regret that.

From the first time that I went to Seattle, Harvey taught me that my thinking is important, that I can contribute, and that I can influence the world. These main points have never left me. He lit a fire in me and gave me a way to understand life and to deal with it. He is gone now, and I am indebted to him. I was liberated by his work. I still am. Harvey, I apologize. Thank you.

33

THE CANYON WHERE THE RIVERS CONVERGE

Wheelchair Rafting and Reflecting

Summer 1986

David Cronenberg's remake of *The Fly* will be released soon, with Jeff Goldblum in the title role.

Two BIG TELEPHONE companies had a contest recently. Each bribed the customers of the other to switch over to its company. After switching back and forth between the two companies six or seven times, I had enough money to pay for a week-long rafting trip down the Green River, a tributary of the Colorado.

Have wheelchair, will travel.

We drive a thousand miles through six states in two days, then sleep, get up, and go down to the river at dawn.

Just before we put in, Lynn, the admiral of our little fleet, gathers everyone together. Lynn is deeply tanned and carries herself like a judo master. There are about twenty of us altogether, including the staff. Lynn is speaking.

"… but if you do fall off the raft, remain calm …"

I consider this advice to be sound.

"… don't panic …"

Even sounder.

"… just relax …"

Would that I could.

"… and float on your back, head up, arms at your sides, feet facing downstream."

I'll just jot that down.

"This will protect your head."

Leaving the rest of me to do what? Fend for itself?

"Listen to your oar boat captain."

Aye, aye.

" If she tells you to get away from the boat, get away from the boat …"

As night follows day.

"… and when she tells you it's safe to get back in the boat …"

Honestly, now. Is any boat ever *really* safe?

"… get back in the boat."

I'll do my bit if you do yours.

We drift, the *café au lait* water moving slowly, lazily spinning the rafts. Around a bend, a whole new vista spreads out before us. Rock walls grow higher on either side as we approach the Gates of Lodore, like an enormous castle with walls made of hardened sediment, thrust up, then cut by relentless water, forming a narrow, curving entrance through which we now wind, far below stone towers and parapets, drifting into the canyon keep.

In the canyon now. Time slows down. For some reason, we are talking more softly, as though we have just entered a cathedral. We pass a small herd of bighorn sheep, grazing on the ledges of the lower canyon wall. A few of them study us. The sound of the moving water, some flies buzzing, the trickle from oars echoing off the rocks. River time, measured by the sun and the water.

It seems like the water is flowing a bit faster now. What's that sound? It's getting louder. Faster. What's that up ahead? Louder. Then the water starts to move very fast, and, hold on! The raft bends and curls as the white-water carries us over and then around a boulder! We are shooting the rapids! The water is roaring now! Hold on tight! There's no turning back! Up and over! The boulders are bigger now. Rushing past. White water rises up and soaks you! There's no going to shore! If you fall in, or if the raft flips, you'll be at the mercy of the rushing water, crashing into giant rocks! Between two boulders! Splash! Here we go! All you can do is hang on! Lay low! Watch out for the rocks! Don't panic!

And we're through.

The roar is behind us. Fading. Then gone. Once again, the current is slow, the river quiet. The raft drifts effortlessly.

At the oars of my raft is Torben, who seems to have baseballs for biceps. In the shade of his floppy hat are massive, carved cheekbones and sunken eyes that match the sky. I am in the bow, facing him.

"I am trained to rescue people who fall overboard," says Torben, dipping one oar to keep the bow pointed downstream.

"Oh," I say, nodding, actually somewhat reassured, still damp from the rapids.

"If they panic and thrash around, I am trained to knock them out, so I can haul them to safety," says Torben, looking at the water.

"Ah," I say, turning my head, hoping he's pulling my leg. He could have said so sooner.

Note to self: stay in the raft.

Later, we row through an eddy to the overnight spot, next to a sandbar. A grasshopper as big as my thumb lands on my armrest, thinks better of it, and leaves. The rock surrounding us changes shape and grows closer as the sun leaves and the light fades.

∼

When I wake up, the morning light is watercolor, splashed over everything.

I crawl out of my sleeping bag and across rocky sand into the shallows of the pool where the water eddies. I turn and sit, weightless. Half-floating. Across the river from me is a rock wall. A bit downstream, a great stone slab as big as a boxcar that has fallen from above rests at the base of the cliff, with one corner submerged in the river.

This canyon measures time differently than the commuters on the Bay Bridge. Its tilted layers are a stack of stone file folders, ordered by age, with the oldest on the bottom. One of the files is full of the fossilized bones of dinosaurs. To these rocks, it's been a split second since Columbus came.

A wiry endodontist from Palo Alto named Geoff helps me put on sunscreen and insect repellent as I sit by the river in my chair, its wheels sunk a couple of inches into the sand.

"Mosquitos haven't been too bad, so far," he says, rubbing the ointment on the back of my neck. "Looks like you got one right here." He pokes me right above my right shoulder blade.

I thank him as he leaves.

∼

On our last full day we were wrestling in a mud hole by the shore. Everybody joined in. It was wonderful.

That night we sat around a campfire. Aromatic smoke on a cool breeze. Fine river grit in our ears and noses. Between our toes. Everyone relaxed and happy. Sparks twirling up in twisting smoke and vanishing. The sound of flowing water and crackling fire. Tired smiles.

I am across the fire from the group, on the sandy patch that has been designated as the stage for the talent show. Tired eyes twinkle in the flickering light as they watch me. I'm sure my beard and hair are sticking out every which way. It's my turn. I tell a story.

"Twenty years ago, I was on the Concorde, bound for Rome, to meet the Pope. I was hungry, so, halfway across Nevada, I headed for the galley. As we passed over Salt Lake City, I went to what I thought was a refrigerator to get myself a peanut butter and jelly sandwich. But when I opened the door, *BOOOOM!* We broke the sound barrier, and, *WHOOOOSH!* I was sucked out of the plane, flew through the air, and then, *SPLASH!* I landed in the Green River at the foot of Steamboat Rock. Needless to say, I've never been the same since. If you look for me, at about this time every year, you'll find me returning to that spot in the river."

The campfire is out now, cold. I think everyone is asleep. I can't see the moon, but its light is on the rock face across the river. Then the moonlight disappears, and I look up and watch as the sky above us fills with stars.

Living in the city, I forgot how many stars there are. With all the city's lights, I could only see a small fraction of the stars that I can see here, sparkling overhead on a clear summer night. It's like they've been waiting for me to come back and are happy to see me again.

Do you see the Little Bear, Ursa Minor? Do you see the tail? The last star on the tail is the North Star. It doesn't move. All of the other stars rotate around it. The North Star is the axle, the hub, and all of the other stars are spinning around it like they're attached to a giant wheel of fortune. It alone stands fast. Shakespeare even had Julius Caesar boast that he was "as constant as the northern star." It's so poetic, like the zodiac itself. Everything else moves, everything else changes, nothing else stays the same, only this one star. The lodestar. The North Star.

If only it were so simple.

The North Star's more formal name is Polaris, because it is directly over the north pole. But it isn't. It's off by almost a degree.

And it's supposed to stay in one place. But it doesn't. It moves around. It moves around a lot. In fact, the night before Julius Caesar crossed the Rubicon, Polaris was nowhere near the pole position.

The truth is, the earth wobbles as it spins, the way a top does when it's losing steam. And the axis line, drawn through the poles, points all over the place, over time. In history, several different stars have occupied the pole position. And one cycle of the earth's wobble lasts 26 thousand years.

The light from Polaris that's hitting my retina right now left home about 300 years ago. Polaris is really three stars that orbit around each other in an awkward gravitational folk dance. The biggest of the three changes in brightness at odd intervals. It pulses. Not only that, it's been getting brighter gradually for centuries.

So, tell me: where is the constancy in all of that?

Even if the North Star *were* fixed in place, straight over the pole, it would only be fixed when viewed from just the right point in space at just the right time. Any appearance of constancy would be more illusion than coincidence. In this universe, there is no such thing as a permanently fixed place or time.

Here, stars explode while other stars are born, galaxies collide, and suns are swallowed whole by black holes that themselves may give birth to new universes. Time expands, contracts, and becomes imaginary. Here, nothing is constant except the speed of light. And even that may be a maybe.

This universe is not a music box, with neat little gears within gears, turning slowly, plunking out "The Blue Danube" as some cosmic spring gradually unwinds. This universe is a jumble of deep silence and simultaneous melodies, played to different rhythms, some to no rhythm at all, and some themes are atonal and come screaming from a far corner of the galaxy, like Jimi Hendrix at Monterey.

This paradoxical universe may be more like me than thee.

I'm really tired.

Tomorrow, we drive home.

34
WRITING THE WORLD

How, What, and Why I Write

Late 1987

Glasnost.

〜

I AM A WRITER.

I am writing, or thinking about writing, all the time. For the last 20 years, I've written something almost every day. I write about my life. One day, people will read what I have written, and say, "Oh, yes."

My writing style is, in part, the result of my early decision to perfect the "One-Fingered Typist" method, employing the Smith Corona electric typewriter, with auto-return, as my instrument of choice. This method is very popular among people who only have one finger that is up for the task of typing. In my case, that finger is my left index finger, the most cooperative of all my fingers. It obeys my commands. It is a good little soldier.

Compared to the drumroll speeds achieved by accomplished ten-fingered typists, the one-fingered method is very slow. It is slower still for me because that relatively compliant finger is attached to a relatively less compliant left arm that is itself attached to a torso subject to unforeseeable jerks, some of which score pretty high on the dystonic Richter scale.

All of this affects my style in three ways. First, my output of typographical errors is prolific, Dylanesque. Second, because it takes me so long to type a word, I am inclined to choose my words carefully, as I must when I speak. Third, there are many time-consuming writing conventions that I respectfully choose to ignore.

While the first point explains itself, the second, which seems obvious at first glance, has at least one aspect that isn't readily apparent. The third will need even more explanation.

To that second point, then. When choosing words, the one-fingered typist must consider many variables.

The standard typewriter keyboard, called QWERTY, was designed to allow ten-fingered typists to type quickly without tangling up the type-bars, the metal arms that hold the typeface bits. Wouldn't it be an amazing coincidence if this placement of keys also helped those of us who use the one-fingered method? Would it be surprising to learn that it doesn't?

As it is, I find myself choosing which word to use based on the number, sequence, and proximity of its component letters rather than making a fetish out of the word's meaning. For example, in a letter to a friend, to express the feeling of being tumbled and crushed in an avalanche of unrealistic social expectations, instead of saying I feel "psychically torn apart" I might say I feel "sad." These last three letters are next-door neighbors on QWERTY.

Don't misunderstand, though. I don't consider this technique to be a personal failing. Far from it. If there were ever a contest to see who could find the shortest rough synonym for any given word with the shortest route between its letters on a keyboard, I would win. Should there ever be a need in corporate America for a master of this admittedly narrow specialty, the job would be mine.

To the third point, regarding writing conventions.

To type the name Al Gore using the One-Fingered Typist method, you have to strike the following keys, one at a time: Caps Lock, A, Caps Lock, L, space bar, Caps Lock, G, Caps Lock, O, R, E.

Using the more popular two-fingered method, you would have a finger free to depress the Shift key while simultaneously striking the A key in order to capitalize the first letter of Mr. Gore's first name. The same would go for the G.

Although the number of keystrokes required for the ten-fingered method is the same as for the two, because each of the ten fingers is hovering like a harrier above its own little burrow of keys, the time that it takes for a given finger to swoop down and strike just the right one can be measured in milliseconds. Using all ten fingers, an expert could probably type the former vice-president's name accurately in about one second, capital letters and all.

Sometimes I type the word "flamingo" really fast, my finger flying all over the keys. It's fun, as long as I don't work too hard at getting every letter exactly right. At times, I feel that I am the Vladimir Horowitz of one-finger typing.

Anyway, I don't use capital letters much, and not because I'm a fan of E. E. Cummings. With all due respect to Mr. Gore, it's just too much trouble and a waste of time. That goes for anything else that requires the shift key. In general, I avoid keystrokes that don't add much to meaning.

There is a fourth element that does more to shape my writing style than mere unidigital typing.

One of the greatest American writers of the 20th century was James Baldwin. He could not have written what he wrote if he had not been Black and gay.

The place that you stand in society determines the angle from which you see it, determines which parts of it are visible to you. Each of us stands in a different place, viewing society from a slightly different angle. But the place where James Baldwin stood was way off to one side. He saw many things that most people couldn't because their view was blocked, or they were too far away, or they were just looking in the wrong direction. His view of society was one that most people had never even glimpsed. His writing revealed his perspective, and that revelation changed the way people see society.

I don't compare myself with James Baldwin except in this one way. I could not have written my articles, essays, and poems were it not for the fact that I am what is called "disabled." More specifically, I could not have written them if I did not have dystonia.

When you are a spastic, you stand way off to one side, away from the crowd. Like Baldwin, you see society from a very different angle than almost everyone else. And not just society, but humanity, even reality itself. You see the backs of things that others only see the fronts of. You see some things that they can't see at all. Things they've never even glimpsed, never even thought about.

Consider. For polite, casual conversation, most people carry around a sampler box of assorted phrases that have been well received by others. Market-tested *bon mots* for small talk. Pleasantries and pointless little anecdotes for every occasion. Put two such people together and the conversation will usually be a friendly little back and forth, consisting entirely of selections from their samplers, never missing a beat. That's not the usual outcome, however, when such a person is face-to-face with me.

He opens his sampler box and selects a phrase that everybody likes to hear, the most popular phrase in the box. I smile, nod, and, in my rich baritone, launch into the first syllable of a perfectly appropriate two-syllable reply. Before I get to the second syllable, however, he has decided that his first choice was wrong, probably because he couldn't find anything resembling my reply on the list of approved responses to his initial selection. His eyes dart around the box, unsure which individually wrapped chunk of chit chat to offer next. He becomes flustered and serves up a phrase usually reserved for small children, then realizes, too late, that I'm not a child. Horrified, he panics, then blurts out something that's not in the box.

I've sat through countless variations of this scenario. People are often so busy wrapping their minds around the fact that they are actually communicating with a real live spastic that they don't have enough intellectual horsepower left over to talk sensibly. You'd think I was a Klingon.

They are so preoccupied by the fact that they are, in fact, communicating with me at all that the content of that communication becomes not only less sensible, but less guarded. Once panic has set in and they've tossed the sampler over their shoulder, the conversations often become quite revealing. It's as though their personal internal censors and propriety guards have gone pub crawling. Seriously, they tell me things normally associated with the confessional or the psychiatrist's couch. Why? What am I, a Klingon shrink?

Maybe they think that being disabled means I am especially discreet. Or maybe, because it's hard for people to understand me, they think their dirty little secret is safe with me. Both these assumptions are dangerous.

Or perhaps they think that I am unusually compassionate, more willing to understand and forgive their trespasses against others. A saint. Or maybe they just figure I'm not in a position to do anything about it.

On the bright side, I feel sure that this effect of dystonia on my world-view has provided me with a more realistic picture of people's internal lives than is usually afforded to anyone who isn't a priest or a shrink. So, if the humanity portrayed in my writing often stands naked, with every scab, scar, bruise, and blemish faithfully reproduced, it is because of the many times that people have politely introduced themselves to me and immediately removed their clothing. Figuratively speaking.

This "disabled confessor" phenomenon is not a direct manifestation of dystonia, but a reaction to it. In fact, most of the phenomena related to dystonia in my social life are in this second order category, in people's reactions to it.

I hope that my writing changes the way people see the world around them, as Baldwin's did. Some things have been changed for the better already, of course, thanks to Baldwin and others before him, but prejudice is still very much alive.

～

Because I am spastic, I am often judged to be mentally deficient. Ironically, it is because I am a spastic that I have had to learn to focus and think with care. I am better able to hear what I'm trying to say and, as a result, am better able to write it. It is because I am a one-fingered typist and type so slowly that I'm not verbose and don't abuse the power of language.

As I live my daily life, cool phrases sometimes come to me, accompanied by a small jolt of pleasure. When the phrase and the feeling come at the same time, I call it a "poetic." I have written lots of them down.

While my output is slow, it is steady. Pages accumulate. It isn't complicated. If you type a page a day, at the end of a year, you have 365 pages. In ten years, thousands. Well, I've been cranking out around a page a day since I was 13. So I have lots of pages.

I wrote for the Ojai paper when I was in high school and wrote the article about my experience with acupuncture when I was at Fairhaven. At Moorpark I wrote a column in the school paper and started up a magazine for disabled liberation, *Complete Elegance,* for the co-counseling community. *Rising Tide,* the newsletter for the disabled community at Solano, was replaced by *Special Effects,* a zine that I started up shortly after the move to Berkeley. Much of what I write now is about creating a culture for disabled people.

I also write letters to people who have the public's attention.

For example, Dewar's Scotch is running an ad campaign called "Dewar's Profiles." Each ad is a one-page glossy resume of a person who drinks Dewar's, complete with a flattering portrait. While there are all kinds of people, they are all both, (a) accomplished professionals and (b) cool. But, if you look carefully, you will notice that not one of them is disabled.

So, using the Dewar ad format, I made a mock-up that features a certain Mr. Neil Marcus, his torso bare, bringing to mind Johnny Weissmuller, who played Tarzan. In the required category, "Latest Accomplishment", is written: "Achieving mobility through public transportation."

I sent the mock-up to Dewar's ad people, gently nudging them in the direction of inclusive advertising. They responded with a nice letter but did not do a "Dewar Profile" of a disabled person. I am waiting.

I have written to Xerox, Samsonite, President Reagan, Celestial Seasonings, and the American Conservatory of Dance, among many others. Pushing. Teasing. Mimicking. Entertaining. Lampooning. Making the case.

My children's book, *The Princess and the Dragon,* reimagines the role of monsters in fairy tales. And princesses in wheelchairs.

My poem that has received the most attention is "Disabled Country."

I've written lots of small things that, taken together, make a pretty tall stack. But I haven't yet written any one thing that I'd call big.

35
STURM UND DRANG
Bringing a Play to Life

1987

**An 18-year-old West German pilot evades Soviet air defenses
and lands in Red Square.
Andy Warhol dies.**

LAST YEAR, MY BROTHER Roger took home a stack of my writing and crafted it into a short dramatic presentation, which he then recorded. Among his many other talents, Roger is a gifted actor. He took the tape to Rod Lathim, the director of Access Theater, a company he founded in Santa Barbara in 1979 to make the stage more inclusive. After one listen, Rod told Roger that he thought there may be something there. When Roger showed him the material he'd mined for the tape, Rod looked through the boxes of poems, letters, anecdotes, and poetics and said he was sure there was a show in there waiting to be born.

They talked it over at length and then Roger called me.

"Neil, we're going to write a play together. What do you say?" I could hear his grin.

"A play?" I answered, "I. Don't. Really. Know. How. That. Would. Work."

"It will be your life's stories, using your words," he said, strategically using the word "your" twice.

A few years before, I had seen Spaulding Grey's one-man show. His life had been shaped into theater. It was impressive. I was wary of a fluff portrayal of disability, but I figured part of my role would be to prevent that. I figured I could keep it real, so I said, "Go for it!"

～

Rod, Roger, and I are at a table outside at a taco place in Santa Barbara, brainstorming titles for the play. For the past six months, they have been huddled over a word processor, writing for hours every day. They checked with me regularly to make sure my original intent was preserved. The script is open on the table in front of me. There are about 24 scenes.

"How about a title from the world of opera?" suggests Roger, carefully monitoring the precariously packed contents of his fish taco. "From Wagner, maybe."

"Or Puccini." says Rod. He plucks a burnt piece of gristle out of his *chimichanga* and grimaces.

"No. From. Nature," I counter, while slowly, carefully moving a *carne asada* burrito mouthward.

Rod takes our empty trays inside the taco place while Roger continues to try out different titles.

"From *The Tempest*, that would be good. Maybe some line by Caliban. Ban, ban, Caliban," he suggests theatrically, gesturing with his taco.

"Yes. But. Not. Tempest. Storm," I redirect as Rod returns.

I want a title for the play that will counter the medicalization of disability. Using an image from nature will help serve as a counterbalance to all the centuries of sterile medical baggage.

"How about, *Readings from the Eye of the Storm?*" suggests Rod.

I think the idea of a storm is right. A force of nature. Swirling energy, filling the sky. Bringing wind and rain. Lightning. A transformational work of art. A cyclone of ideas and insights. Illuminating society. A tornado of words and images that blows across the cultural landscape, overturning long-held assumptions, upending unexamined beliefs, and bending brittle preconceptions until they snap. And all done, of course, with good humor and grace.

"Or maybe, *Readings from the Storm?* says Roger.

And there it was.

"Yeah," I say, "*Storm. Reading.*"

Rod's eyes light up, "Bull's eye!"

Roger laughs.

We start rehearsing tomorrow.

The first scene we work on is from the time I was in my chair on a neighborhood side street and a little girl on a tricycle started riding around me. She warily said "hi" to me several times. I said "hi" back each time. She asked me some innocent questions about whether I could talk, or if I was there to visit. I answered them. Then she asked, "Are you scary?" I said, "No." Her response was to pedal up the front walk to her house as fast as she could, screaming, "Mommy!" Roger plays the little girl. We got him a little trike. He wears a beanie.

The second scene we try out is from a dinner party in Berkeley, where I leapt from my wheelchair and struck an angular, dramatic pose. My host was my friend David Daniels, a poet and artist. He was astounded. He enthusiastically compared my form to the masterpieces of Chinese calligraphy. He said I was a living brush, that I was "total expression."

For the final production, slides of me dancing in a coat festooned with Chinese characters will be projected onto the back of the stage during the scene. Roger plays Daniels.

In the third, I observe that everybody looks at disabled people and everybody looks at movie stars. So, I wonder aloud, "Am I a movie star?"

Then I ask why movie stars like to do charities for disabled kids. Is it because disabled people are living such dramatic lives? After all, society isn't exactly organized to make our lives any less challenging. And disabled people have strong human emotions. We are the living incarnation of bravery, and our presence stirs everybody and everything. Doesn't it follow that in the human drama we are the protagonists, not the victims? Roger and I are decked out as celebs, with sunglasses and hats.

Roger gives voice to my thoughts in the fourth scene:

> I have always maintained that disability is a never-ending quest to achieve perfection. You will read about it at least once a day in the newspaper or as a human-interest story on TV; but they don't quite have the right idea. Disability is not a "brave struggle" or "courage in the face of adversity." Disability is an art. It's an ingenious way to live. Who would ever think of living that way if they weren't disabled?

After a pause, I deliver the punchline. "No one."

~

After the first day of rehearsal, I was still very skeptical. "This? This. Is. A. Play?" I asked Roger. It didn't seem to be like the plays I'd seen. It seemed disjointed somehow. I still didn't get it. We continued rehearsing.

Roger bought a new Nikon and took pictures of me dancing and jumping in the surf. He put together montages of his shots and set them to music. They will be projected on the backdrop to add another dimension to the action on the stage.

As we rehearsed, three hours a day, four days a week, it became clearer to me that what we were doing was going to happen. People were going to get to see into my world.

~

It's a cold night in January in Santa Barbara. I'm staying at Roger's. We've been rehearsing for months. I've never worked this hard before. I have to be very precise. And precision is not my strong suit.

"Okay, take it from the top. Move here; quick. Faster. On that line. No! That one! Face out," says Rod. "Half the audience can't see you. Extend more. Okay, now, once more."

We do several run-throughs of each scene. Down to the smallest detail. We go through the whole play five times. Every scene.

I am working on the dance part, the part inspired by Fred Astaire. Roger says, "This is a first. No one has ever created a dystonic dance before."

We are turning disability into art. It feels right, but the real test will be on opening night, in front of an audience.

~

In February, we move into the Lobero Theater to rehearse. The lights are blinding. I can't even keep my eyes open. We open in less than a month.

It is the morning of the dress rehearsal and I don't want to get out of bed. But if I don't get up, I would lose this chance to get my message out.

The dress rehearsal. I feel like I'm being born again, and it's not an easy birth. I don't think I'll make it to opening night.

But I don't have a choice.

CHILDHOOD

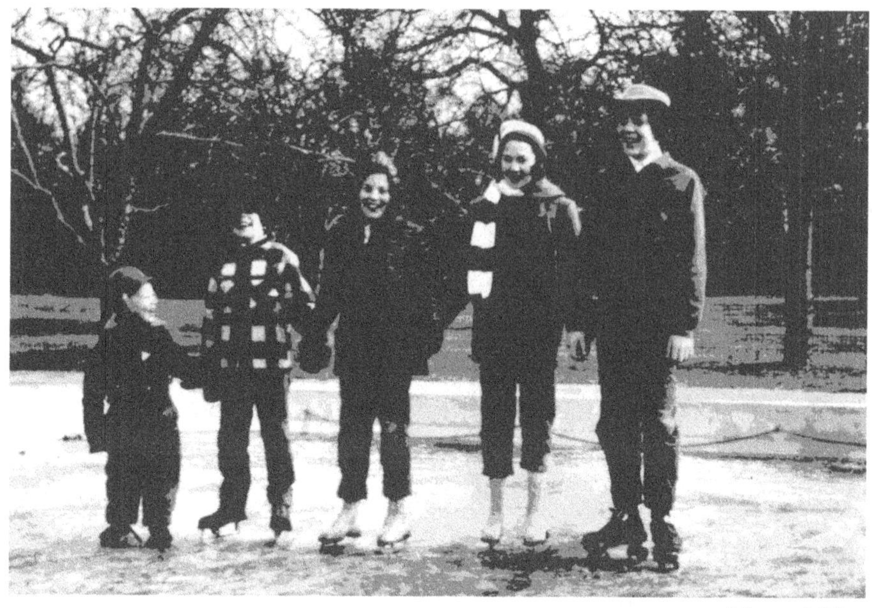

Marcus children
Family photo, 1957

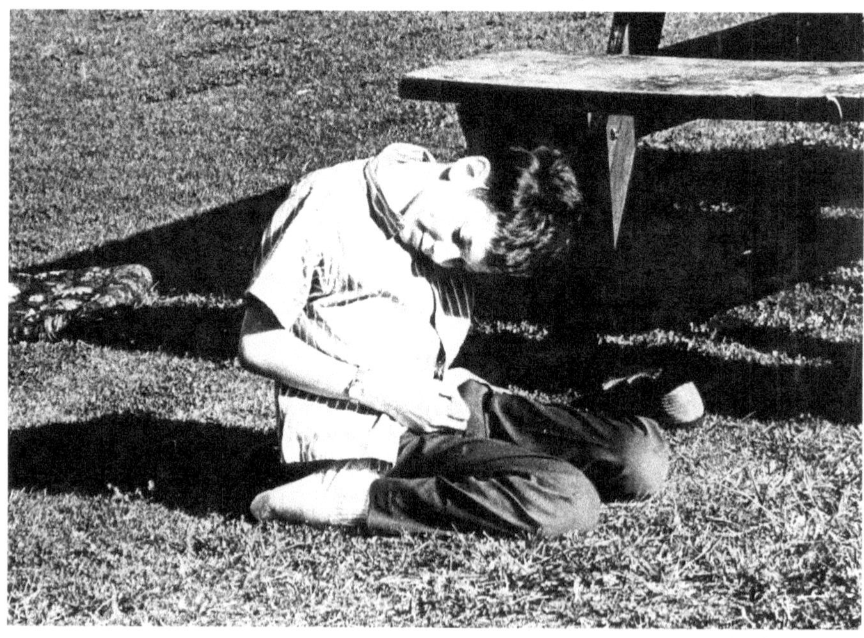

Neil (9 years old)
photo courtesy Roger Marcus

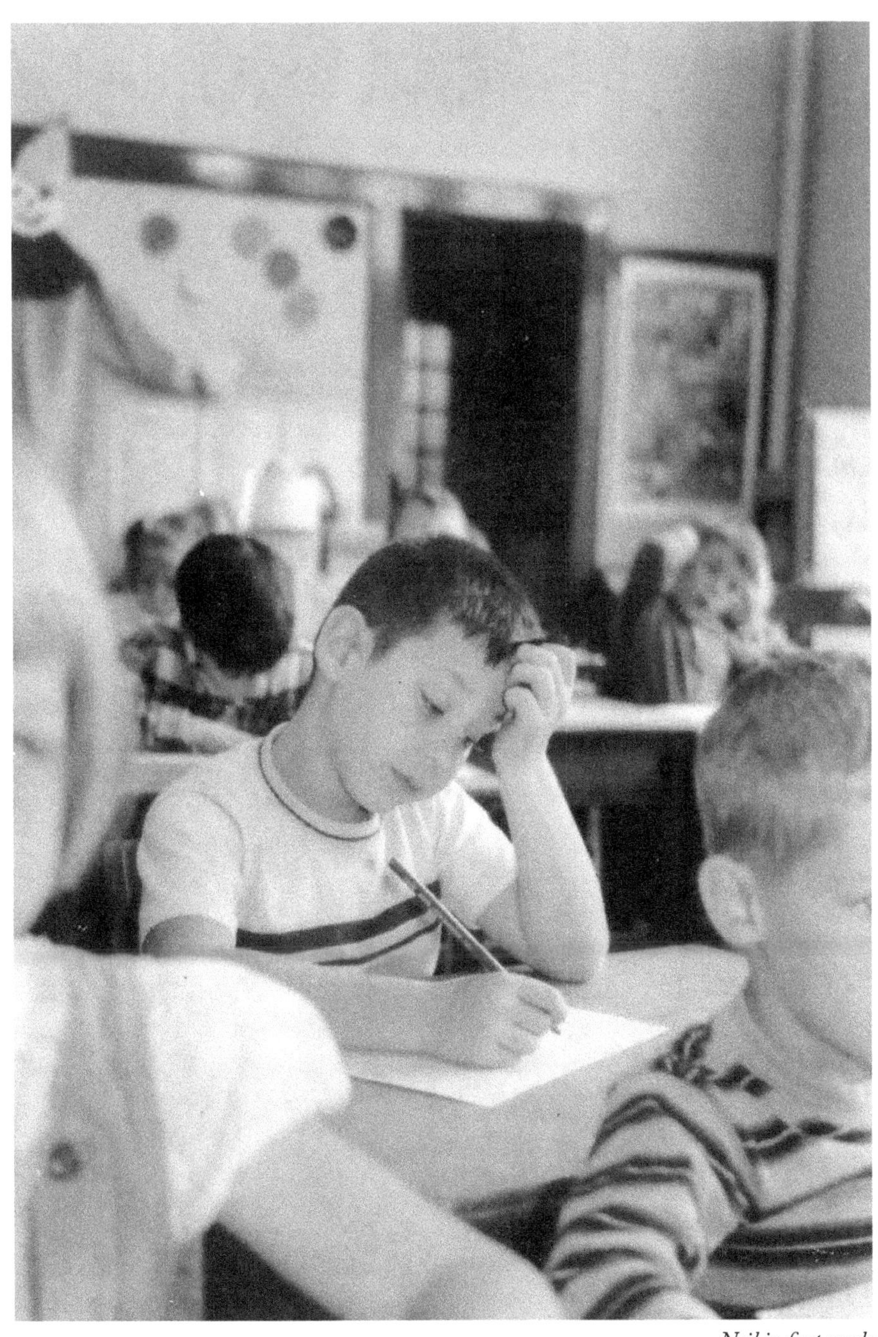

Neil in first grade
Family photo

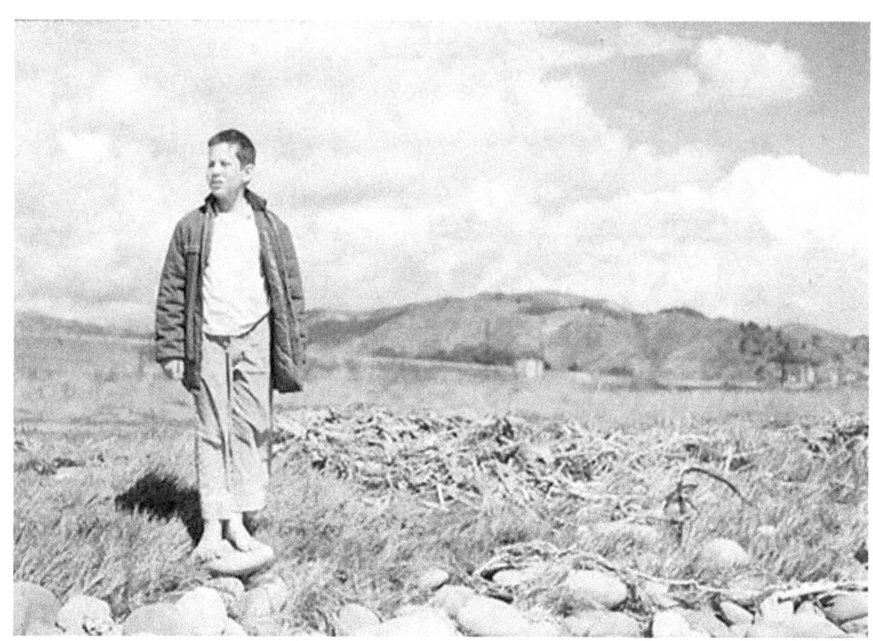

Young Neil
Family photo

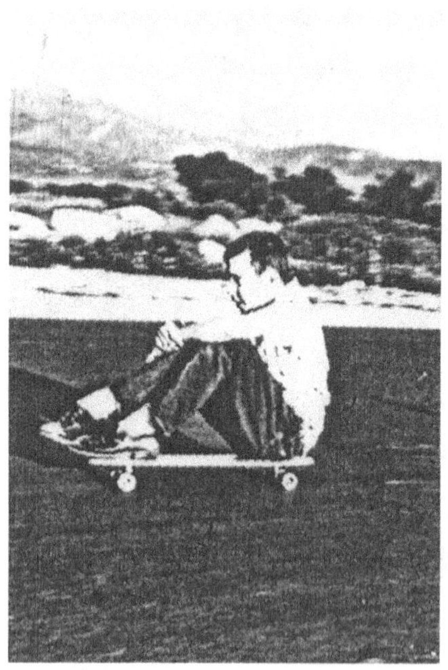

Riding backwards on skateboard
Family photo

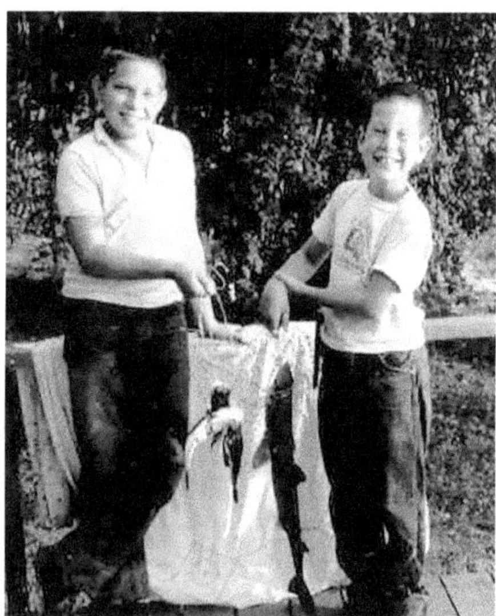

Neil and Roger fishing
Family photo

188

PATIENT

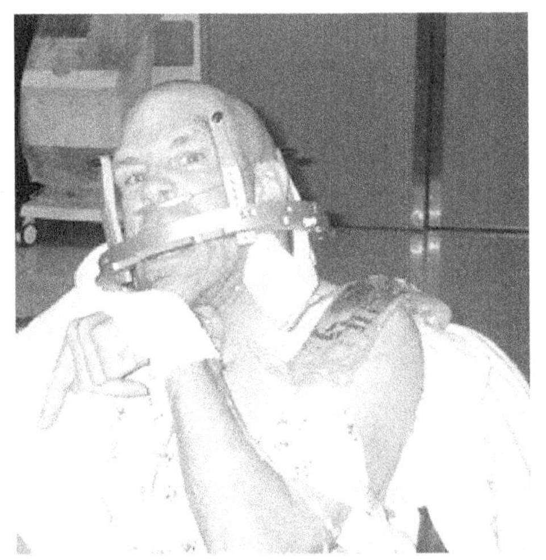

DBS surgery
Family photo

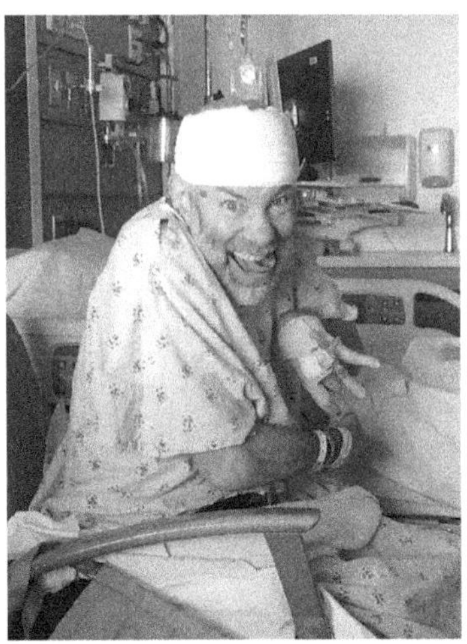

Surgery recovery
Family photo

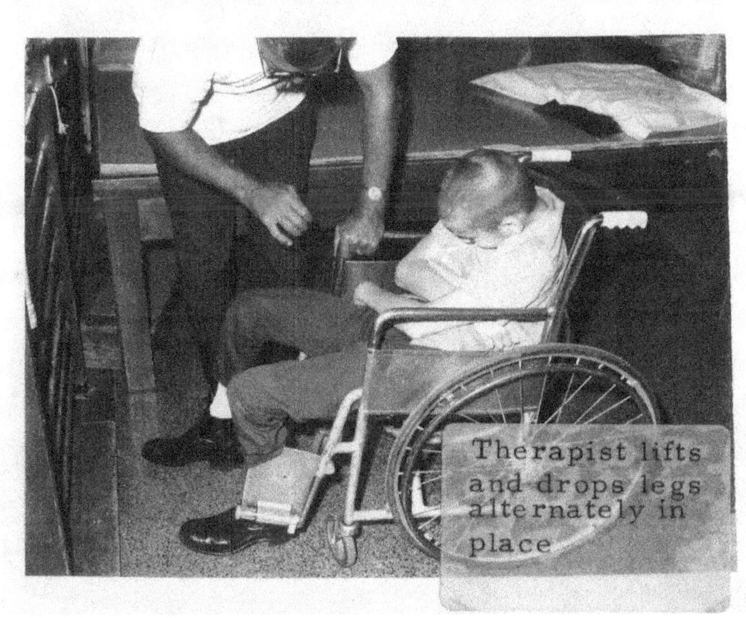

Physical therapy
Family photo

EVERYMAN

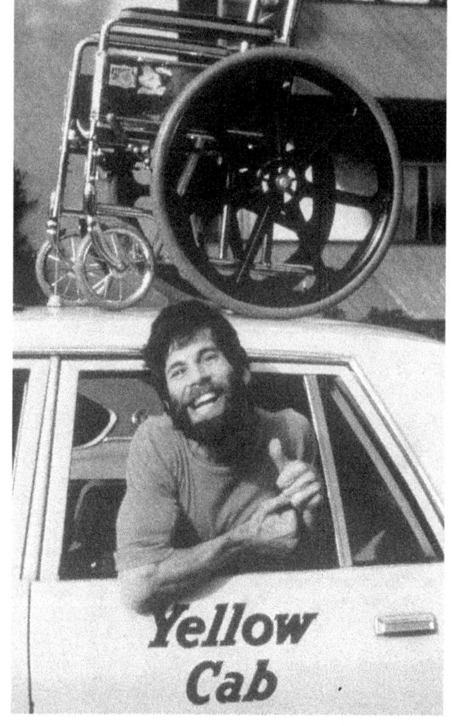

On the move
photo courtesy Rod Lathim

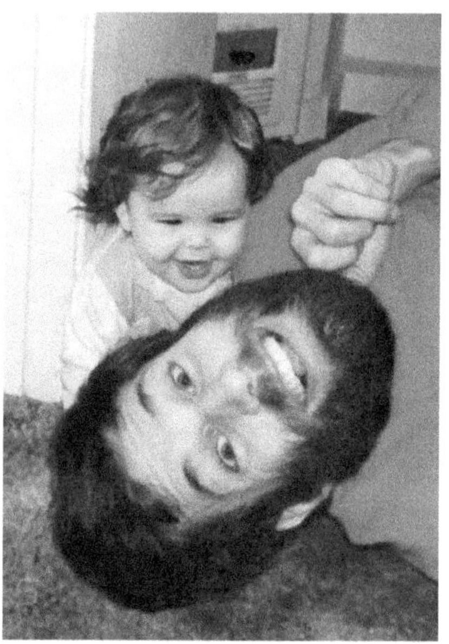

Neil with Emily Hofmann
photo courtesy Mel Hofmann

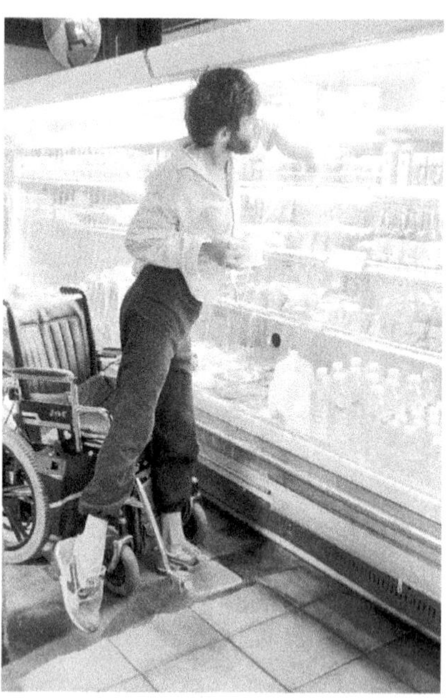

At the grocery store
photo by Brenda Prager

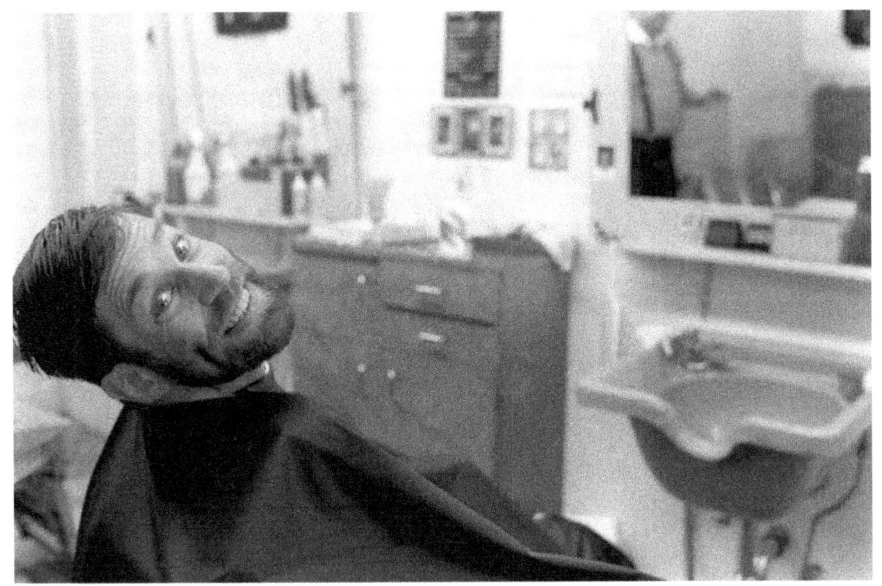

Getting a trim at the barber's shop
photo by Brenda Prager

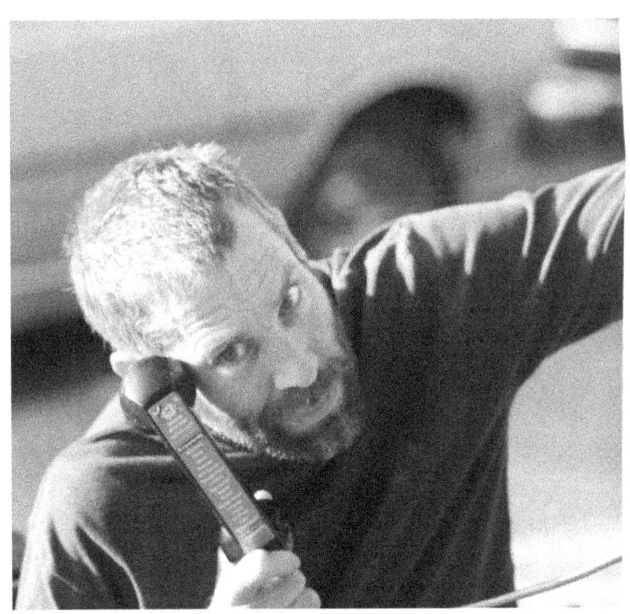

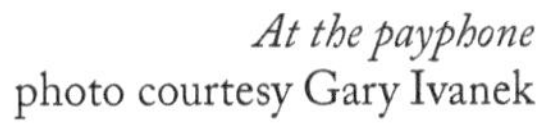

At the payphone
photo courtesy Gary Ivanek

WRITER

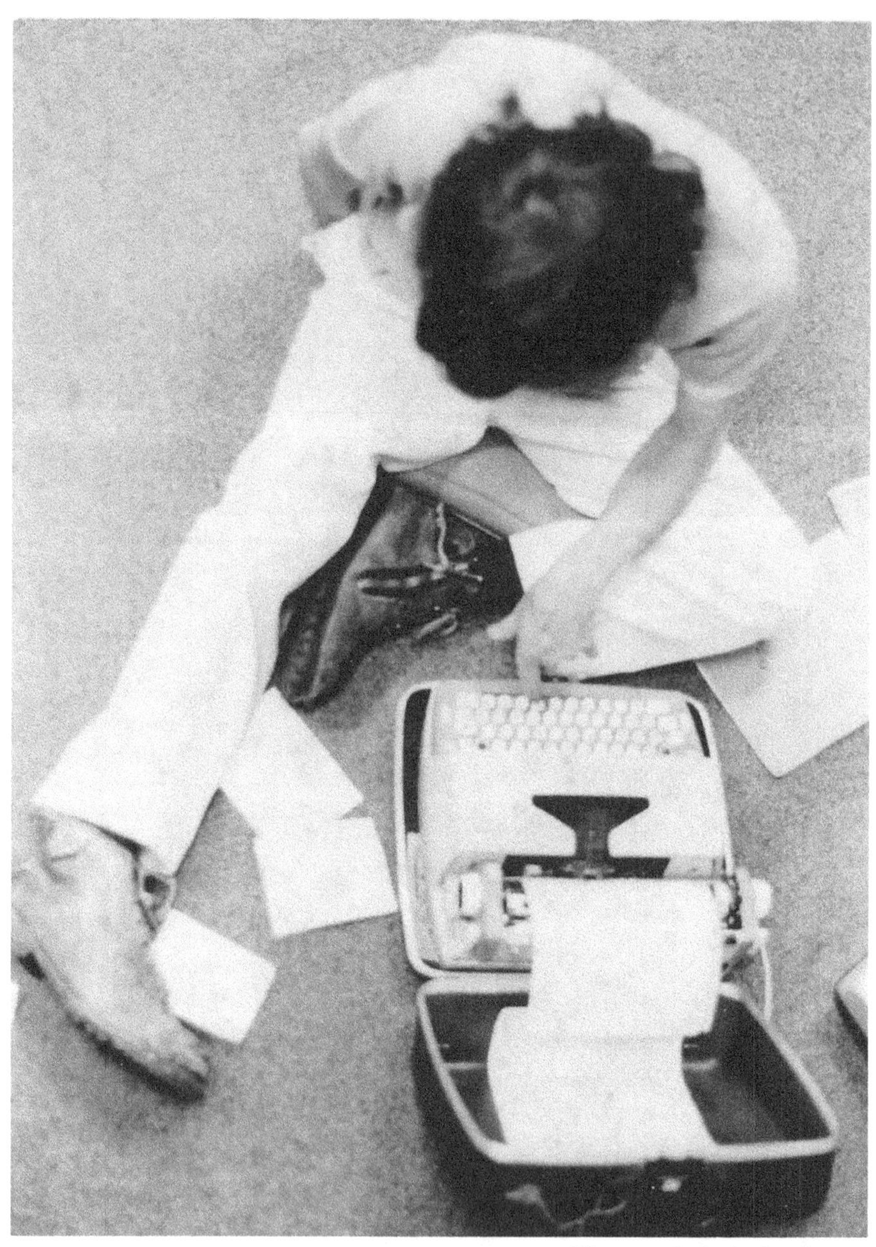

Writing in high school mid–1960s
Family photo

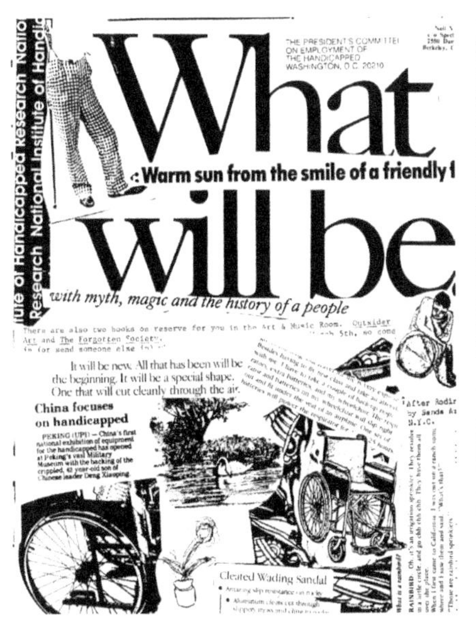
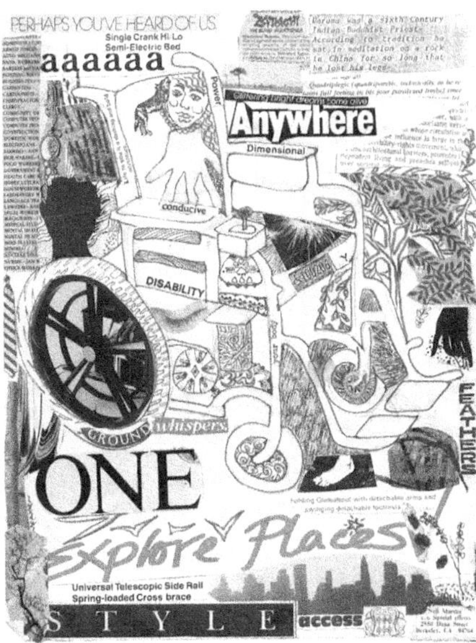

Special Effects zine

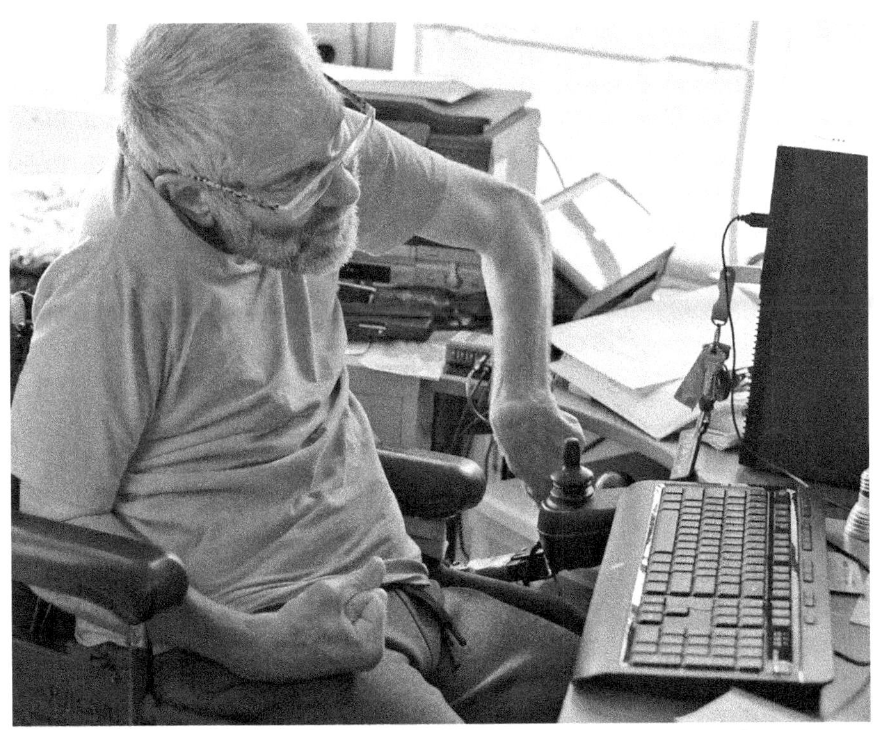

Neil writing, 2018
photo courtesy Mel Hofmann

LETS DANCE. thats the closest ive come to an intelligent response
to the question ,'how can i best be of help getting you from here
to there.'

when i took science in the fifth grade it was in a new building
that had special tables with gas nozzels on them which we never
used. our teacher was also the gym instructor and we gave him lots
of trouble...i didnt,i was 'good' ..but i remember he was always
trying to control our group.
there were cages of white rats all around the room.i remember they
were always having babies.i remember that and i remember their
water bottles which were always empty and i used to go around
during class lectures and fill them. they used to drink and
drink.i used to think it was so cruel for them to be without
water.
i remember the time a goat was castrated.
i remember i didnt have to study too hard cuz i already knew a lot
about evolution.
when i was in third grade my brother gave me a
book about life in a pond.i also got a microscope for christmas.

people often tell me i have a lot of courage. especially people
who meet me for the first time.
i never know what they are talking about....me?courage?im just
living my life. yesterday i felt like i could not go on.i felt
paralyzing fear flowing in my veins. it was affecting my mind;my
will to live.i felt lost in it.my body was freaking out too.
should i go out to eat..no its too hard.should i eat in..no youve
been in all day ..you need to get out.but maybe itd be best to
learn to stay in..no ,thats like death...but so is going out...and
love is that way too..should i call someone...yes.no.its too
hard.and with all this other stuff,its hard to be mr. charming
date ..forget it.but you need it.
hmmmmm. is this what courage is for?

by the next day ,i got over it . i woke up with the terrible
feeling gone.i wrote some letters.went shopping.went to a disabled
peoples rehersal of the nutcracker .called paul and made a
shrimp beet salad for dinner. paul came and brought lettuce.he was
scared because he thought he had left his stove on so he left

Diary entry, 1987

194

ADVOCATE

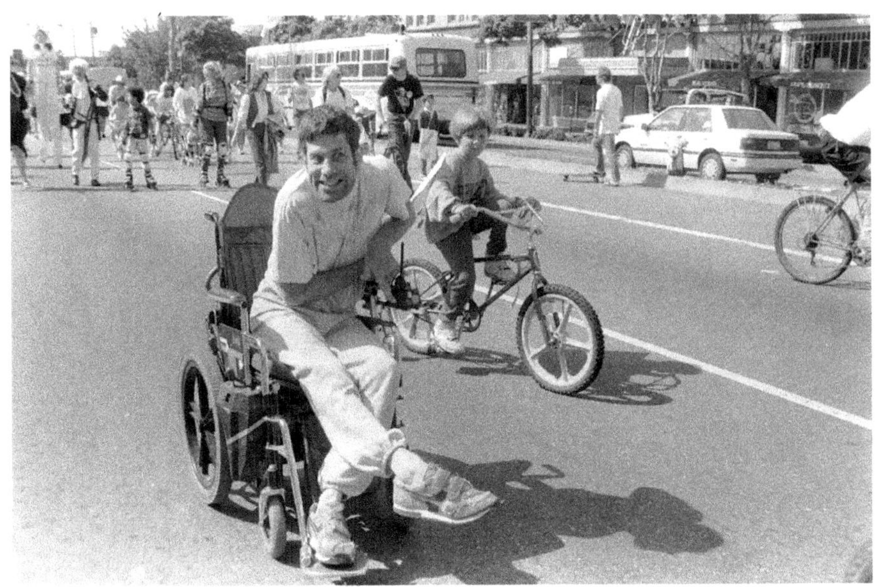

Neil in a march
photo by Brenda Prager

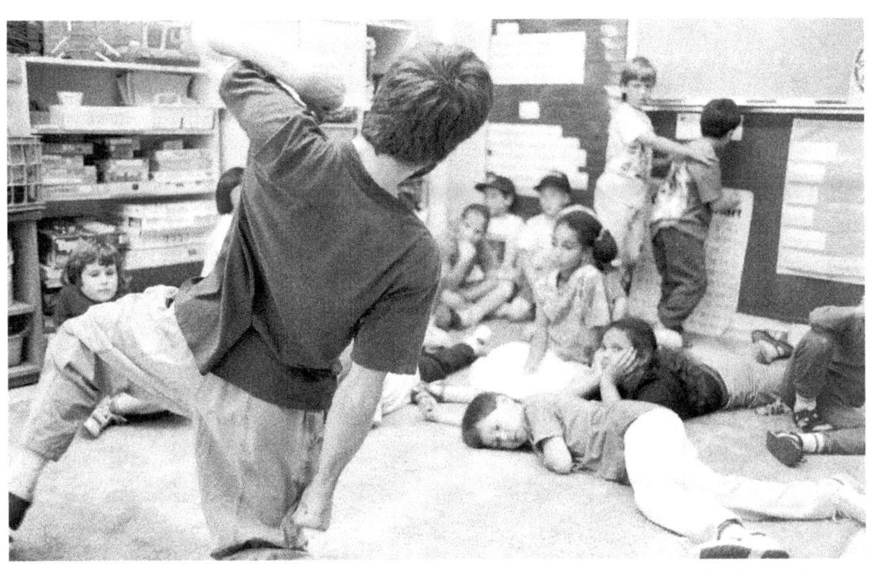

Neil in a classroom
photo by Brenda Prager

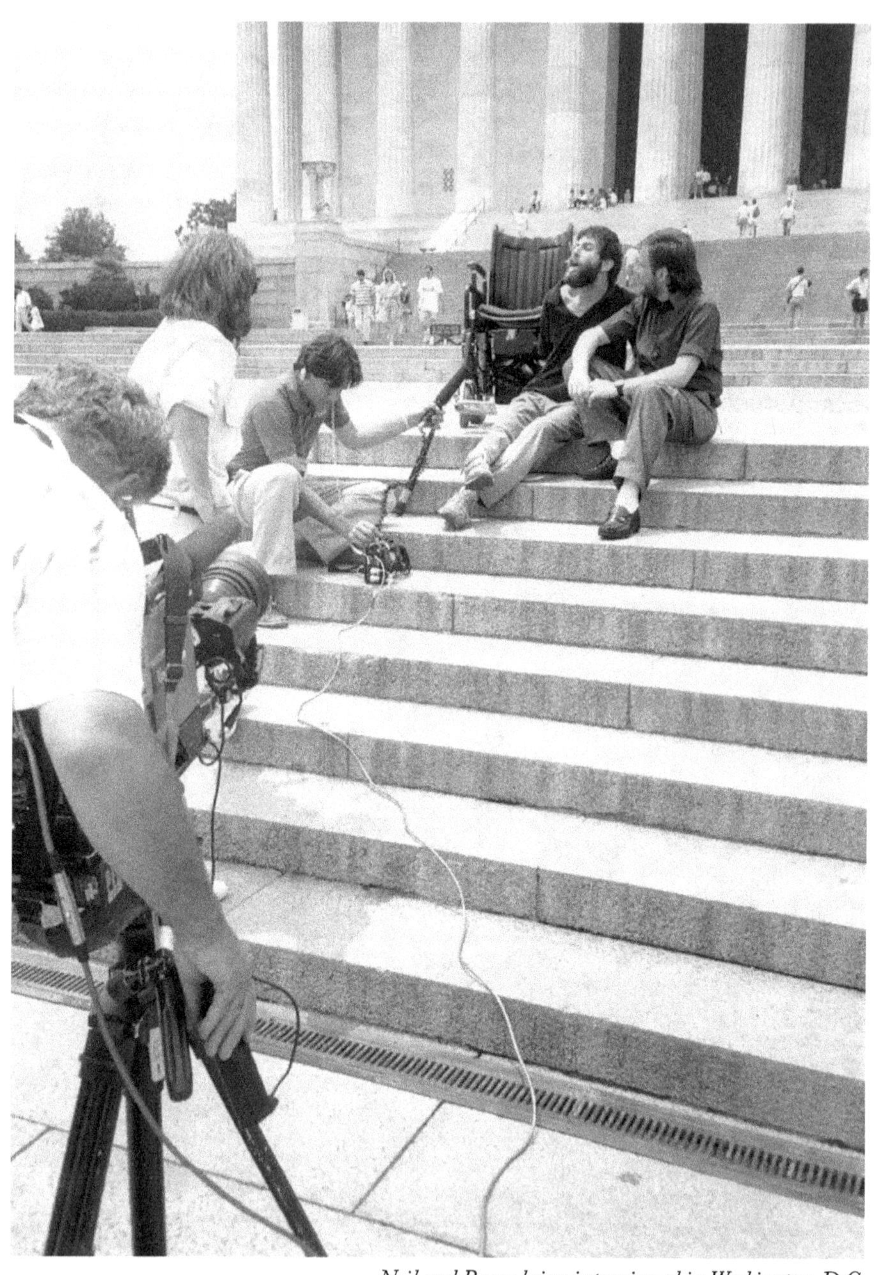

Neil and Roger being interviewed in Washington, D.C.
photo courtesy Rod Lathim

Actor

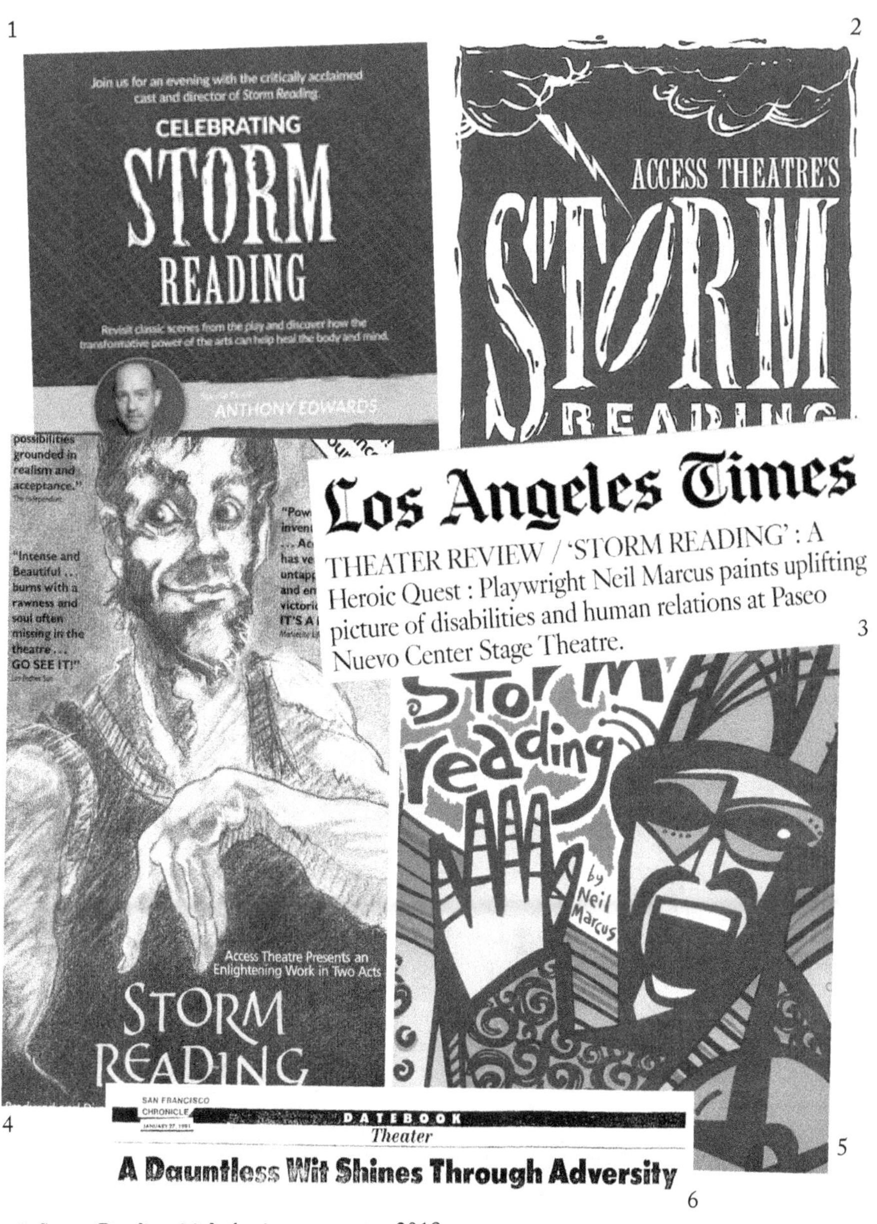

1. *Storm Reading 30th Anniversary poster*, 2018
2. *Storm Reading poster*, 1989, design by Jeannie Sprecher
3. *L.A. Times Headline Review*, 1991
4. *Original Storm Reading poster*, 1988, design by Grace Hodgson
5. *Storm Reading poster for Manchester, England*
6. *San Francisco Chronicle Review*, 1991

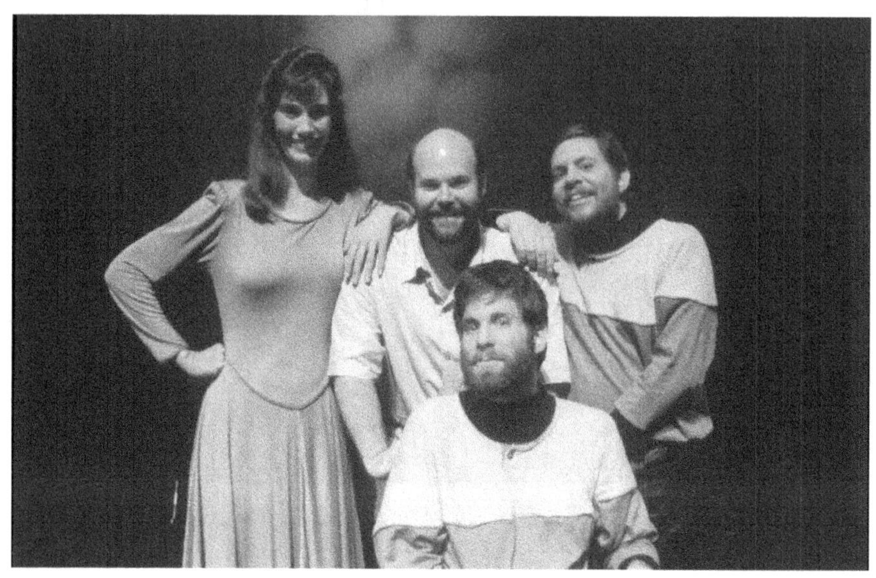

*Storm Reading Original Cast l. to r., Kathryn Voice, producer
and director Rod Lathim, Roger Marcus, and Neil Marcus*
photo courtesy Access Theatre

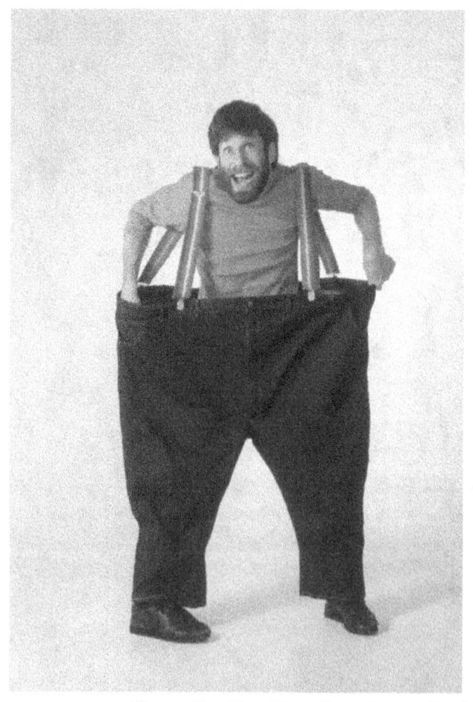

Storm Reading "Rainbow Suspenders"
photo courtesty Access Theatre

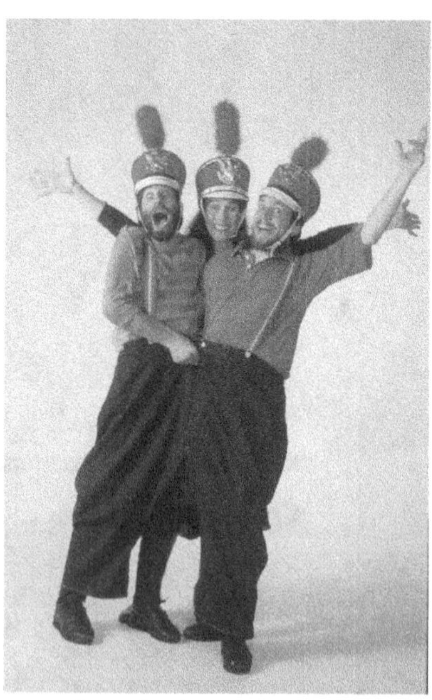

Storm Reading "Rainbow Suspenders"
photo courtesty Access Theatre

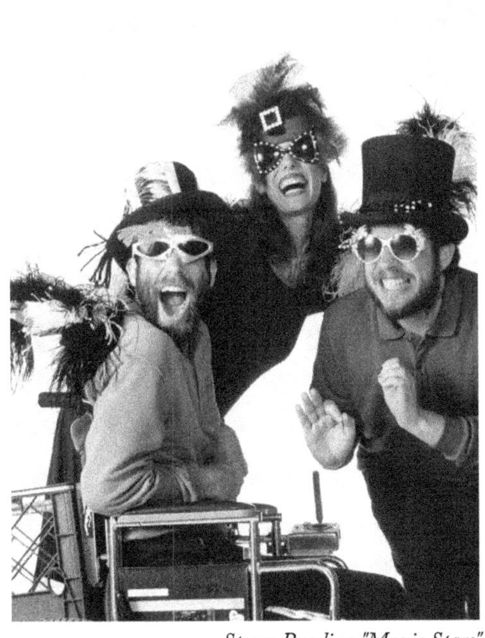

Storm Reading "Movie Stars"
photo courtesy Access Theatre

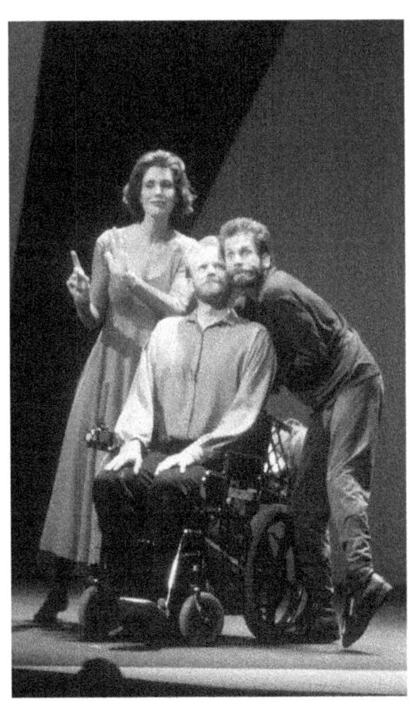

*Storm Reading, Kathryn,
Matthew, and Neil*
photo courtesy Access Theatre

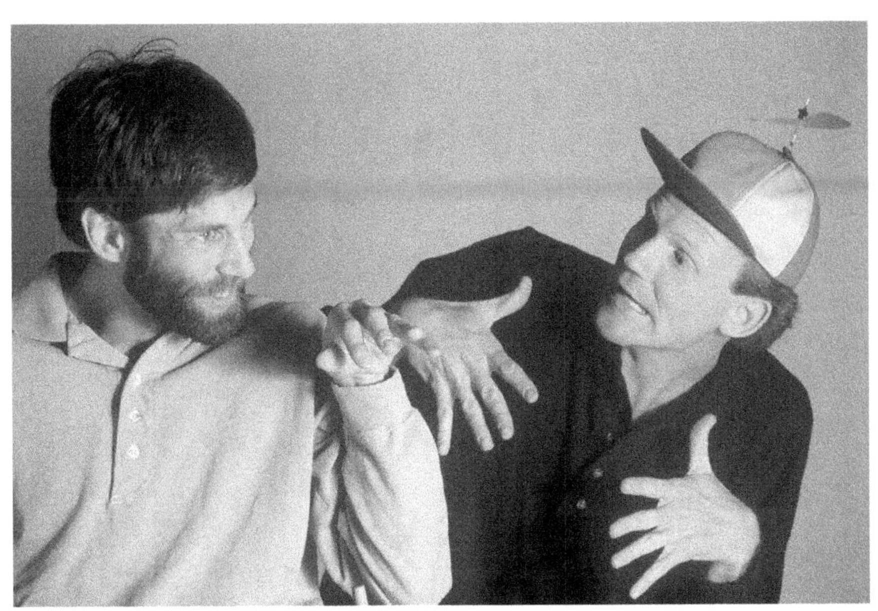

Storm Reading, Neil and Matthew Ingersoll
photo courtesy Access Theatre

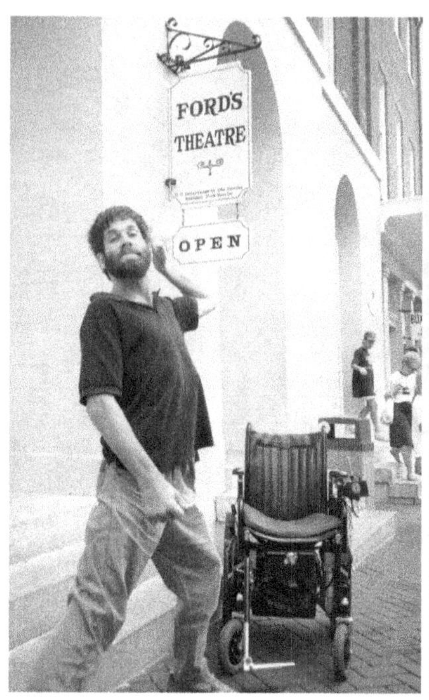

Neil at Ford's Theatre for performance
of Storm Reading
photo courtesy Rod Lathim

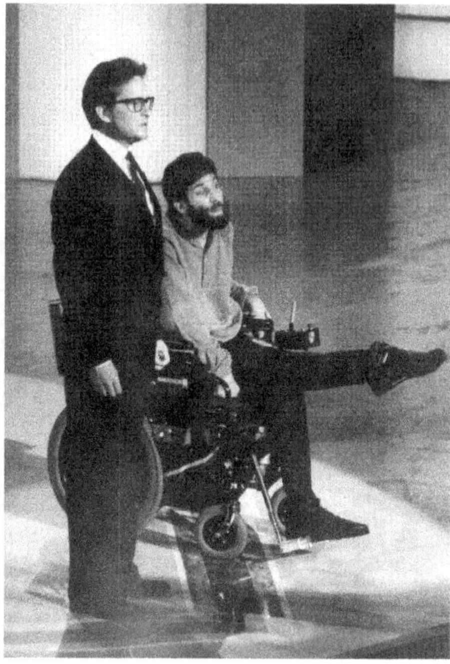

Neil with Michael Douglas
at the Kennedy Center
photo courtesy Rod Lathim

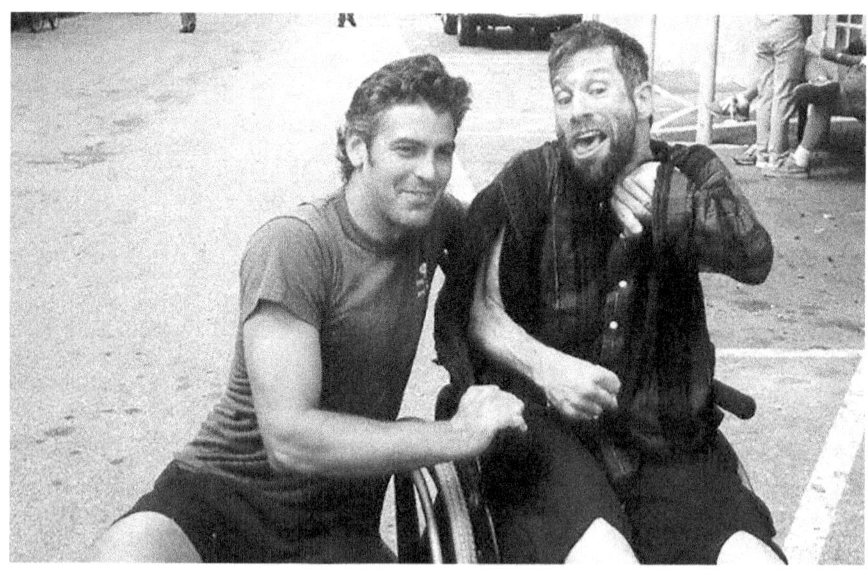

Neil with George Clooney on ER lot
photo courtesy Rod Lathim

DANCER

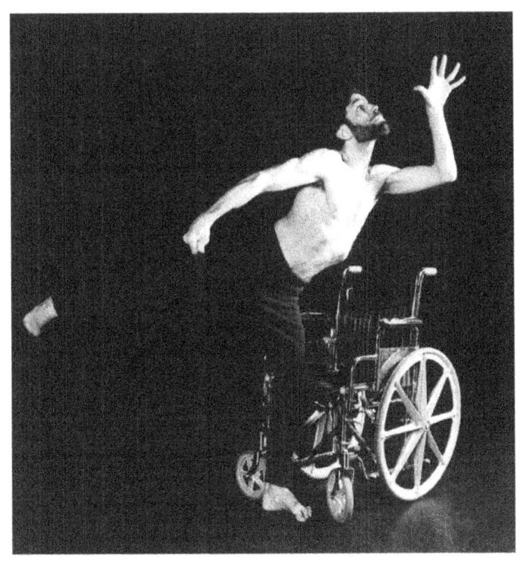

Photo
courtesy Susan Jorgensen

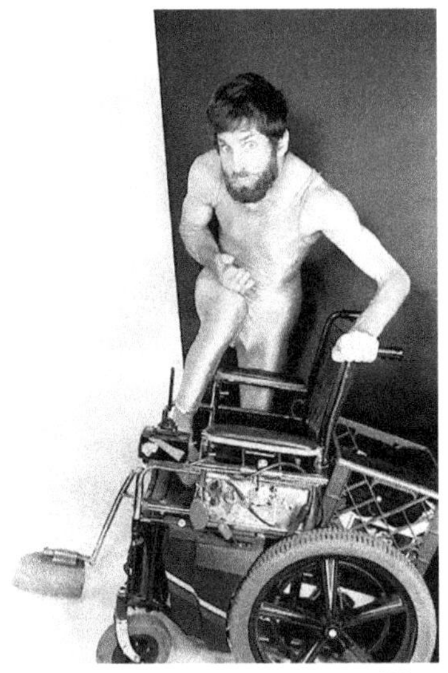

Photo
photo by Brenda Prager

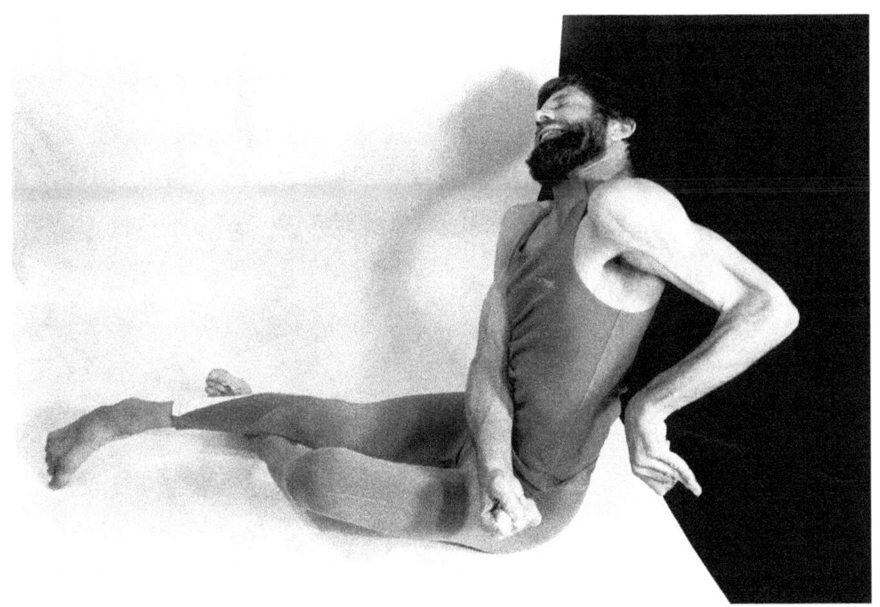

Photo
photo by Brenda Prager

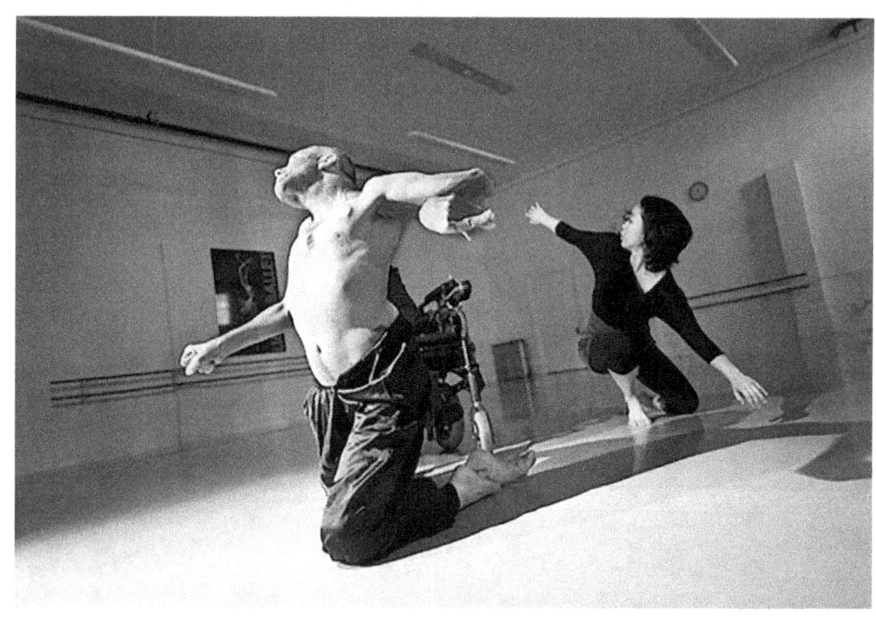

Water Burns Sun, butoh dance video, an Olimpias Production, dir. Petra Kuppers.
Production still by Keira Heu-Jwyn Chang

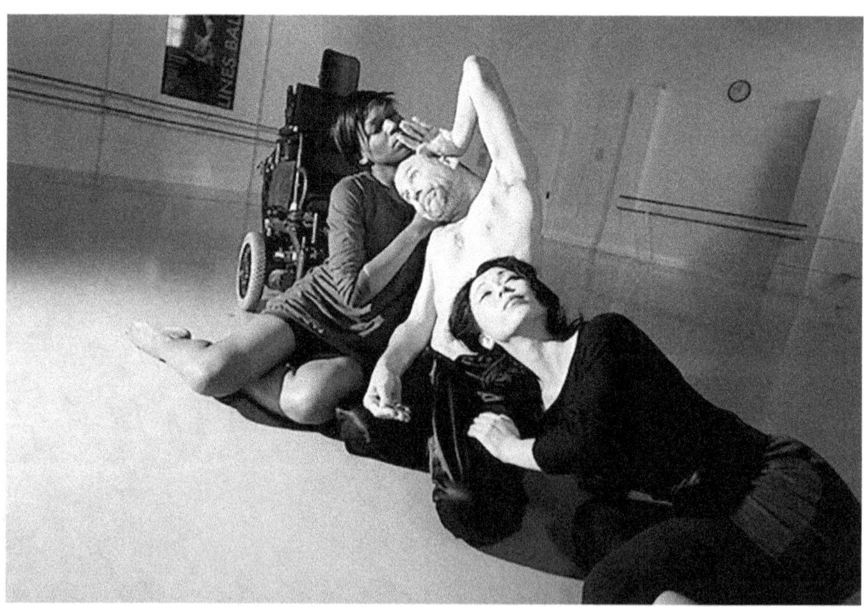

Water Burns Sun, butoh dance video, an Olimpias Production, dir. Petra Kuppers.
Production still by Keira Heu-Jwyn Chang

ARTIST

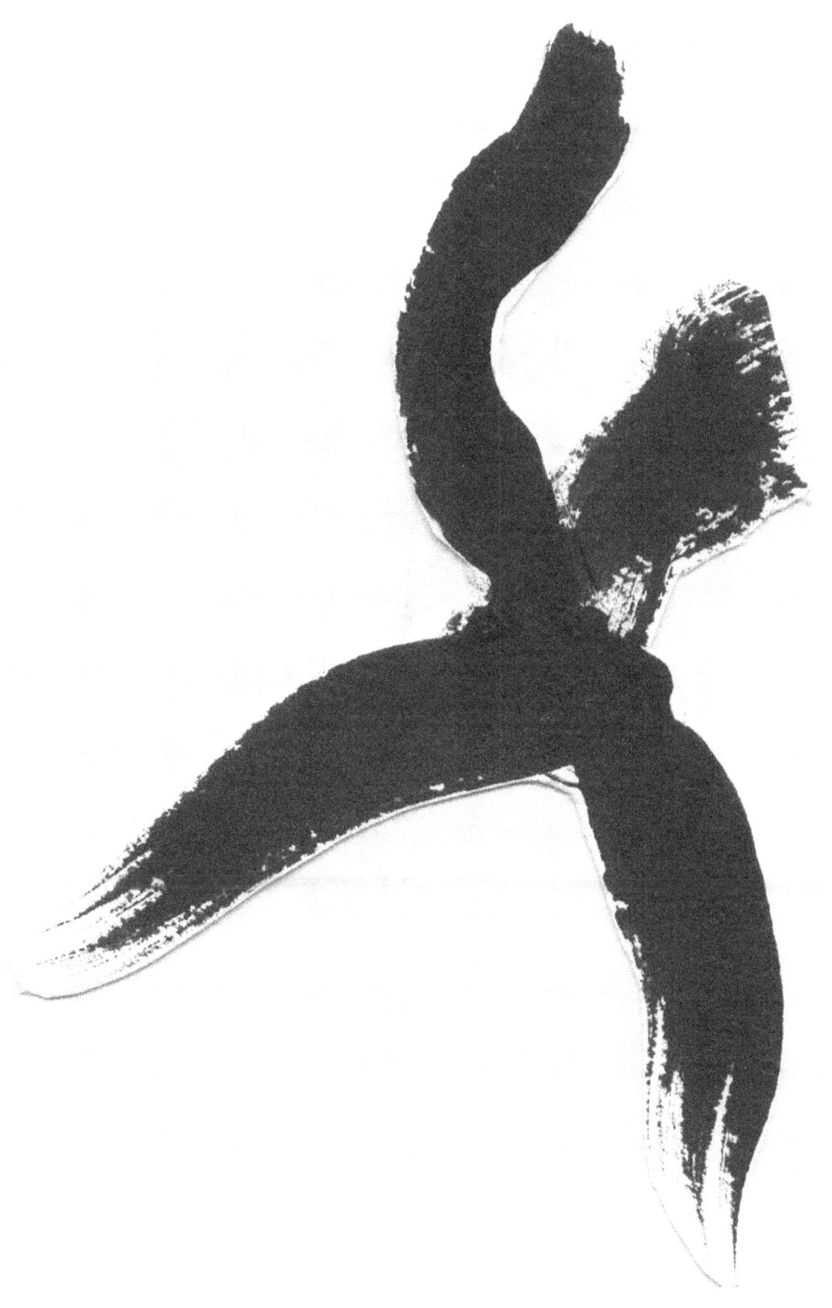

"Flying" calligraphy
by Neil Marcus

203

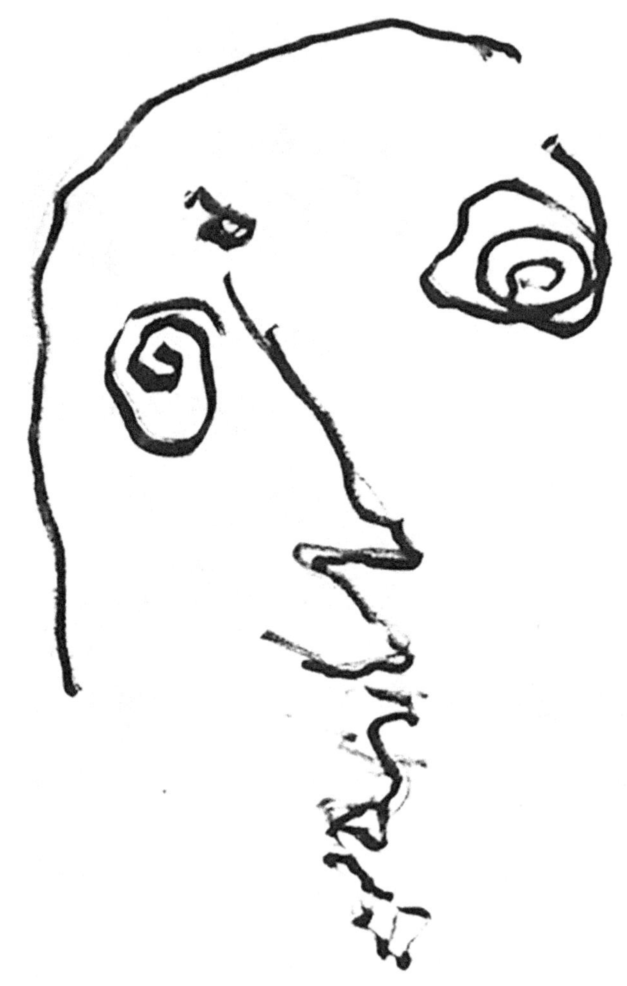

"Face"
by Neil Marcus

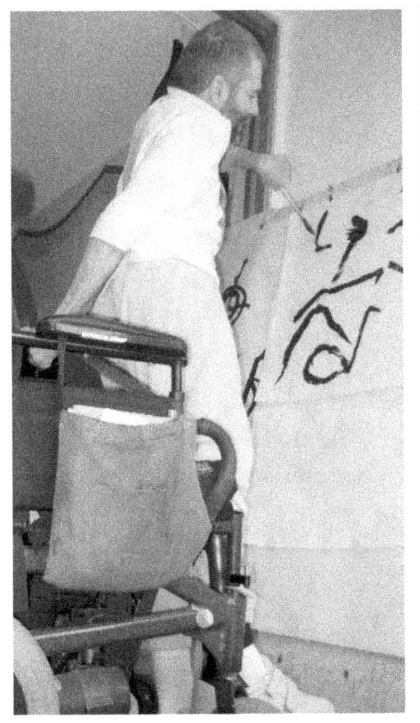

Neil painting
photo courtesy Gary Ivanek

Neil painting
photo courtesy Gary Ivanek

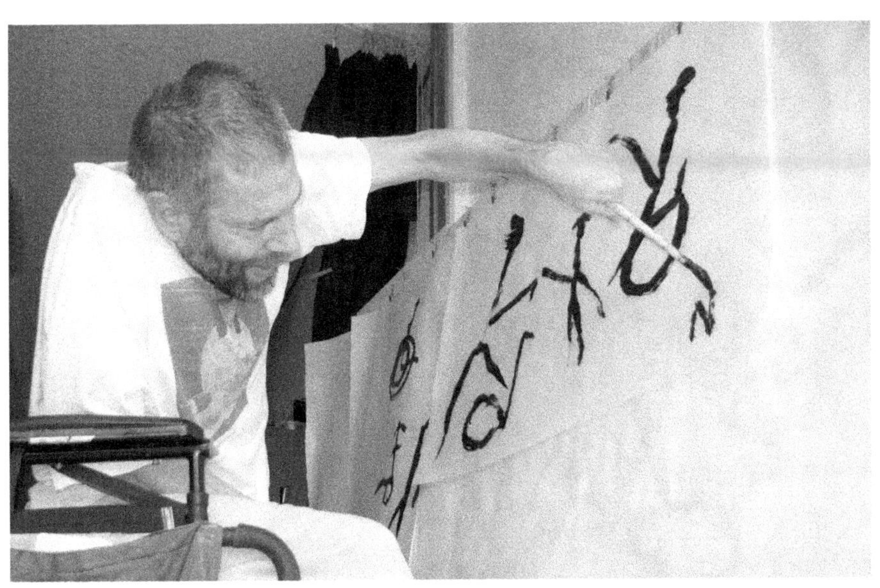

Neil painting
photo courtesy Gary Ivanek

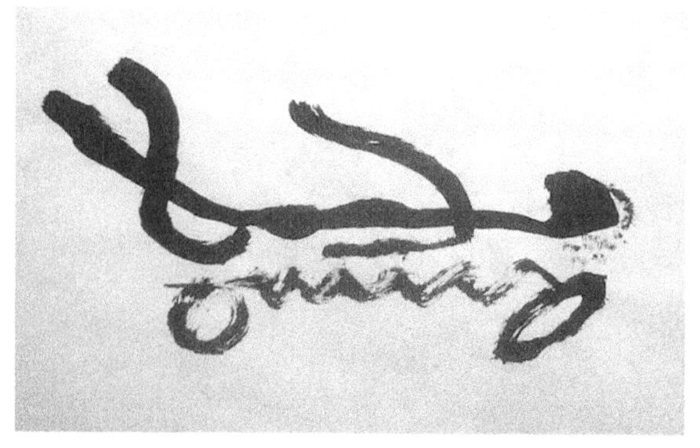

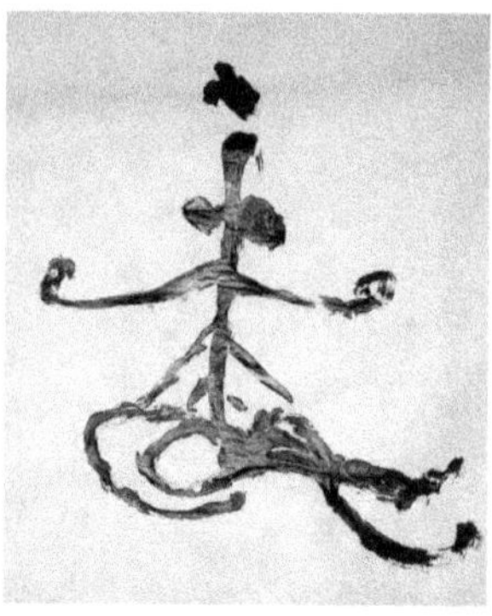

Untitled
by Neil Marcus

In a Wheelchair
Calligraphy by Neil Marcus

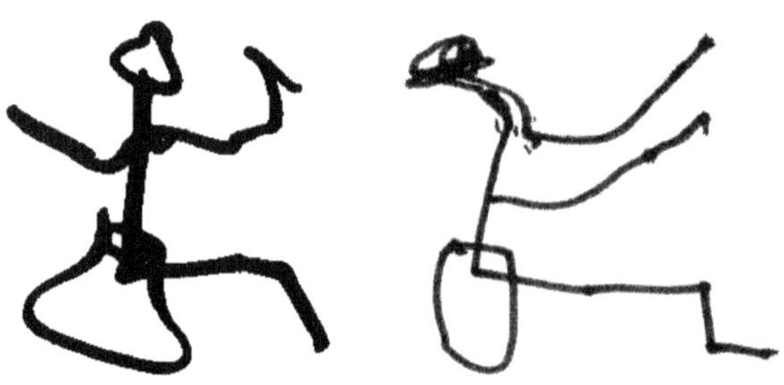

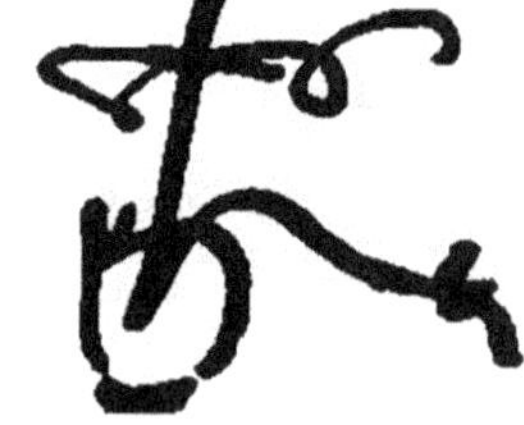

In a Wheelchair
Calligraphy by Neil Marcus

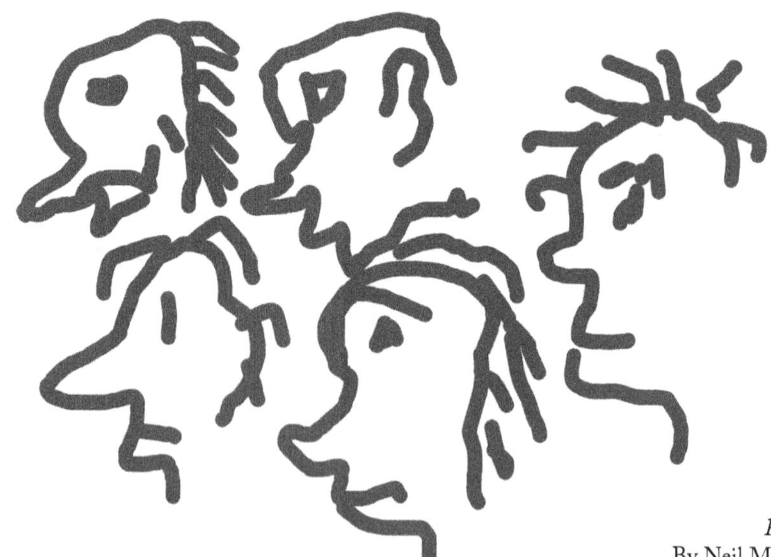

People
By Neil Marcus

36
PEEKING FROM BEHIND THE CURTAIN

Facing the World

March 4, 1988

Later this month, Michael Douglas will win the People's Choice Award
for Best Movie Actor.

The Soviet Union is on the brink of collapse.

A CENTURY AGO, SANTA Barbara decided to unify the architecture of the city
in the Spanish Colonial Revival style. So, in 1923, the Lobero Theatre was
lovingly rebuilt, with hand-troweled, white stucco walls and an unglazed,
terracotta clay tile roof. Igor Stravinsky and Vladimir Horowitz have
performed here. On this stage tonight? *Storm Reading.*

I do an interview with a local TV station. There is a final dress rehearsal.
I learn what it's like to wear makeup under the lights. Costumes, dressing
rooms, the green room. All this is new. Everybody says, "Break a leg."

My god, it's about to happen. It's opening night.

I'm on in five minutes.

I wait in the wings, out of the view of the audience.

Dressed in black.

Unexpectedly, my mind carries me back to Silver Pines Camp. I am an eight-year-old boy, on the lake, sailing in a dinghy, alone, far from shore. Swimming, my legs, my arms, my body, below the surface, hidden, slowly veering off course. Then I'm back in school. Limping behind the bushes between classes. Sitting in the back row. Pulling my cloak of invisibility closer around me. All the shyness, the shame, the fear. Then I see myself as a college freshman, screwing up the courage to eat in the cafeteria. I've felt all this before. The desire to hide.

But now I am a 34-year-old man, and the Lobero Theater is sold out!

Get a grip. It's just stage fright, I tell myself. Everyone says it is a perfectly normal reaction when you stand in front of your fellow human beings and say, "Look at me. Here I am."

Well, I'm not normal, and I'm not perfect. But I've beaten this fear before. And I will beat it now. I extend my right index finger, my good little soldier, and touch the arm of my wheelchair. Wrapped there, under two layers of cellophane packing tape, is the penny my dad put on the tracks when I went to Silver Pines Camp. The one he called my good luck piece. Then I realize that I'm smiling and I smile more broadly as a result.

My whole family is here. My friends are here. People I have known all my life are here. So are lots of strangers. Remember Fess Parker's promise? Daniel Boone? The tuxedo? He's a no-show.

"Two minutes, Neil," the stagehand whispers.

I manage to nod. The house lights are dimming.

Be calm. Acting on stage is like a giant bio-feedback loop. The energy goes back and forth. It builds and builds. Breathe deeply. Nothing feeds the loop like uncertainty. The goal is to relax and act. Focus. I am not Ralph

Ellison's *Invisible Man.* I am out here for all to see. For all to hear. I feel sweat on my forehead, my pulse racing. Steady. If the fear of disability is largely the result of ignorance, well then, I am going to shine a very bright light on that ignorance tonight. Focus.

The murmuring from the audience grows softer, then sputters. Three voices, then two.

The house is dark now.

The stage is dark.

The audience is silent.

I'm on.

I roll on unseen from stage right in my trusty power chair. I stop at a black wooden cube, about two feet high, and get on top of it. Still in the dark, I crouch low atop the cube.

Then, *pop!* Colorful abstract shapes are projected onto the screen behind me just as soft, slow music begins. I rise slowly. As the music builds in intensity and volume, as the images become more complex, layer upon layer, I unfurl my limbs and extend my spine, rising, first to one knee, and, as the music gathers strength, and reaches its crescendo, I stand, a dark shadow, stark against abstract layers of bright color. I raise my arms, like a titan, a champion in his moment of triumph. I hold the pose. Then, blink! The music ends abruptly in a twinkling sound, like falling tinsel, at the precise moment that the theater becomes completely dark.

The darkness fills with the sound of clapping.

In the midst of the applause, I get back in my chair and go to front center stage. As soon as I get there, *pop!* The spotlight blinds me and makes the audience, not me, silent and invisible. It's showtime.

I speak.

～

"People are watching me. They're watching me all the time. They're watching me even when they're pretending not to watch me. They're watching me to see how well I do this thing called human."

I could deliver these lines, but it would take too long and a significant portion of the audience would turn to the person in the next seat and whisper, "What did he say?"

The solution to the problem is found in theatrical crafting. Throughout the play, whenever I have to give a speech like the one at the opening, I deliver the first sentence or two, and Roger joins me on stage, saying the same lines, as I sort of taper off. It's the acting equivalent of the hand-off in a 400-meter relay. For it to work, it must be done adroitly, and timed perfectly. Roger is really good at it. When done just right, the audience simply accepts Roger as my voice. I think it helps that we are brothers and look somewhat alike. In most scenes, my lines are short, and I deliver them myself.

Kathryn Voice, an experienced professional actress, completes our little cast. She has the dual duty of playing roles in many scenes while simultaneously signing the dialogue of all the characters. Her classical grace as she navigates the stage breaks the usual rules for ASL signers and contrasts nicely with my somewhat edgier style.

At the end of our opening night, the three of us stand together at center stage. The audience is on its feet. People are laughing and smiling, some with tears in their eyes. I think they had expected a sad disability pity story, but after the curtain calls, as they exit the theater, I hear them still chattering excitedly. They are still smiling. It's like everyone's heart opened up.

The play is over. I've done it. I've made it through. I've shared my life. They're all cheering wildly. I've moved the world.

Five curtain calls.

"A knock-out!"

That's what the paper says, anyway. I'm at my brother's, at the breakfast table, reading the *Santa Barbara News-Press*, while chomping on granola and strawberries. It seems the reviewer approved of *Storm Reading*.

"Dazzling, profound, ingenious."

This is very good.

Determined to catch this small wave, Rod arranges for a one-night stand of *Storm Reading* at the 1300-seat Doolittle Theater in Hollywood, paid for with help from Michael Douglas and David Seltzer, both Santa Barbara residents and patrons of Access Theatre. Invitations are sent to all the executives in the entertainment industry.

The idea is simple. If the big shots like it, they'll tell others and interest will grow. If there's enough interest, bookings will pour in. That's the idea, anyway.

It's like placing a big bet in roulette. If it doesn't work, we sleep in a camper. In the snow.

37

A Shindig on Hollywood Blvd

A Gala Performance for Movie Moguls

Early summer 1988
The Red Army will soon withdraw from Afghanistan.

~

ON THE MORNING OF THE performance, I drive with my family to Hollywood. We find the Doolittle Theater on Vine Street, but all the parking spots nearby are taken, so we have to unload our stuff a block and a half away and haul it up the sidewalk. Everybody has bags and is pulling things with handles.

A union guy named Hank unlocks the main entrance doors, leads us through the dimly lit lobby, and opens the door to a dark room. He throws a switch, and *pow!* A huge pink and green room with row after row of bright recessed lights appears. A thick pink fuzzy carpet runs from wall to wall. All the makeup tables and counters are black marble. The furniture is chrome and black leather. The air conditioning is blasting. Hank speaks.

"This was Lily Tomlin's dressing room when she was doing *The Search for Signs of Intelligent Life in the Universe*. More than 200 performances. All right here."

He is clearly proud of his part in the production.

It's noon. We go check into the hotel. We've got to have lunch, then be back by two. In costume, in makeup, ready for filming by the local NBC crew. We also have to do a run through of all the lighting cues. Lots to do. Showtime tonight. Pressure. We make it back at two sharp.

"Hi, I'm Bill Anderson, the house carpenter. Pleased to meet you. I've heard so many good things about you. Good luck!"

Then Bill reads us the riot act about making sure the union guys do all the work. We're not to move anything, get anything, or change anything ourselves. We must ask a union guy to do everything for us.

"Don't do anything yourself. We're the union."

The union crew is off until three.

The NBC crew shows up and tapes a wireless mic to my back. We start to shoot a scene, and the mic keeps jabbing me in the middle of my back. I go into spasm overdrive. The pain, the performance pressure, and the overall stress of the day are too much. I start really spazzing out.

Roger, who's in the scene with me, notices, looks a bit alarmed, and says, "What's wrong?"

I now look like a Greco-Roman wrestling coach demonstrating a self-administered submission hold. Roger studies my pose, his agitation growing, and says, "This is not how we rehearsed it!"

He's right, of course.

We do a three-hour run through. Every step is cued with lights through a computer. Everyone is on edge. We break at six for dinner. I'm exhausted. And scared. It's two hours till curtain. NBC is filming. I'm getting dressed again. It's seven. It's an hour before curtain.

This just isn't possible. My body is as tight as it gets. A sailor's knot. The combination of stress, anxiety, exhaustion, and conflict is like Led Zeppelin blasting throughout my central nervous system. If I have to fight my way through this for the opening, I might die.

I could take a muscle relaxant. It would reduce the tension, the tightness. But would it affect my acting, rob me of my energy, my vitality? What to do? What would Lily Tomlin do?

I take it.

I eat noodles and a tuna fish sandwich. The local NBC crew films our preparations. "Just ignore us. Act like we're not here."

Okay. Here I am pretending to ignore that I'm being filmed by NBC.

Curtain's at eight. It's eight.

Rod talks to us.

"Just go out there and enjoy yourself. Throw away your cares. Relax. You're ready."

Easy for him to say.

I roll out onto the darkened stage.

Afterward, there is a standing ovation. We do questions and answers from the stage. People line up in front of the stage to greet us. There's a reception in the lobby. A guy invites us to perform in the Soviet Union.

"Yes. In Moscow!" Lots of hugs and kisses

"You were great!" "Thank you!"

Everyone is smiling, some through tears. We have a party in the hotel.

Maybe it's okay for me to feel like I'm going to die on stage. Maybe it's okay for me to be weak, to stumble, trip, and fall. This play is no longer about my life. Now, it is my life. And this is what my life is like. Really. Why shouldn't people see it all?

Mistake? How can I make a mistake when everything I do is authentically me? So I can't get a line out. So what? I fall. Great fall, Neil! Whatever I do is, by definition, a valid part of the theater experience. Maybe this is unlike any theater ever done before. This is the theater of reality. The theater of life itself.

I find this thought liberating.

～

Standing ovations. Rave reviews. Congratulations for one and all.

And then.

Nothing.

38

ONE LEVEL HIGHER

On Tour and Network TV

Summer 1988

Radio Shack introduces the Tandy 1000 SL computer.

***Rain Man* is on location in Kentucky.**

～

ROD WAITED BY THE phone, pen in hand, ready to juggle booking requests for *Storm Reading*.

One week. Two weeks. Four. Five.

It was beginning to look like the storm had fizzled out.

Then a theatrical booking agency took us under its wing and booked us for a few engagements in Oregon. After that first small tour, a few more dates were booked. Then a few more trickled in. After each performance of *Storm Reading*, the audience would leave and tell other people about the show. The word spread. Soon, booking requests were pouring in.

People started to ask me for my autograph. You've heard of celebrities who resent the intrusion? Not me. For so much of my life I pretended to be invisible and people pretended not to see me. They avoided even being near me. I was ashamed and they were afraid. Now they walk up on the street and ask me about myself.

I'm making up for lost time.

You want my autograph? Sure!

~

We flew into Denver this morning. I'm in a hotel in Boulder, Colorado, resting, getting ready for tonight's show.

Earlier today I did a live interview for the local TV morning talk show. The interview went okay, but my hostess made the fairly common mistake of assuming that because I sometimes need a little help, I must be a child. She even talked to me in a higher-pitched voice than she was using with everyone else, and it was sort of sing-songy. The fact that she was interviewing me because I am acting in a play that is based on my own writing might have tipped her off. One would have thought that my full and luxuriant beard might have helped her guess my age.

At the end of the show, she walked over to me, still talking baby talk, telling me how much she *loved* meeting me, and then she grabbed my face with both hands and kissed me, patting my cheeks as she pulled away. And then she patted me on the head. On camera!

To her credit, the questions were quite good. I didn't even have to trot out my usual dog and pony show about overcoming a disability. To be honest though, I think it unlikely that she was the one who wrote the questions.

She meant well. She probably just reached into her sampler, couldn't decide which *bon-bon* was appropriate, and grabbed the one she usually reserves for her two-year-old niece.

Ah, well. She just didn't know any better. No harm done. Must rest. Show tonight.

~

It's about a half hour till the show. I'm in the shadows, offstage. I can see Rod out front, talking to a group of about six deaf kids as Kathryn signs for him. A girl says she's never seen a show with an ASL interpreter before. Not on TV, not on a stage. Another kid looks interested, but hesitant. Rod coaxes him in a friendly way. The kid signs that his name is Martín and asks Rod where he learned to sign. I can tell that Martín is uncomfortable just being here. It draws attention to his difference. I sigh. I know the feeling, Martín. Curtain up in fifteen minutes.

≈

We now know which scenes are the biggest crowd-pleasers. We've tinkered with them based on the audience response. We add and drop lines, and monitor timing, volume, pauses, sequence, looking for the best dramatic effect.

No two nights are the same, of course. I never know when my right leg will decide it's time for a big goose step, or when my neck will decide that my head has been on vacation long enough. And every now and again, I inadvertently let fly with a bit of saliva. Sorry, Kathryn.

The most popular scene is the one where I'm at a Burger King. I'm on one side of the stage, ordering at the drive-through. Roger, wearing headphones, is on the other side. I try to order, but he can't understand me. The audience can't either. I try again. No good. Finally, I go slow, syllable-by-syllable, as clearly as I can. Sloth talk.

Roger hesitantly repeats it back to me. "A cheeseburger? Vanilla shake? And onion rings?"

I shout, "Yeah!" He joins in and then we both sing, "Have it your way, at Burger King!" That's the jingle from their ad.

This Denver audience loves it. They're still clapping as Roger comes back on wearing a white lab coat. Now he's a goofy professor. The Jerry Lewis version. Squeaky nasal voice. Funny glasses. He introduces his lecture: "Spasticity in Movie Theaters." That's my cue. I roll up next to him, hop out of my chair, and stand next to him, balanced on my left leg, using him for support.

The scene makes fun of the medicalization of disability with a series of gags. At the end, the professor gives me, the "good specimen," a little treat for being a good, compliant subject. As I take the treat, I bite Roger's thumb. The audience howls.

～

Tonight, everything clicked. I feel like I'm the master of the stage. After the last scene, the stage goes dark, the house lights go on, and the applause is loud. Then the audience stands. I see lots of people crying, but not because they're sad. They're smiling and laughing. They're moved. I can see it in their eyes. They're astounded.

Roger leans over to me and, raising his voice, says, "Before *Storm Reading* you were using a pea shooter to try to change the world, now you have a cannon!"

Then Rod and the three of us sit in chairs lined up right at the front of the stage to talk with the audience. I'm still uncomfortable doing this.

Martín is sitting in the fourth row with his hand half-way up. I know about that half-way thing. Rod calls on him, Kathryn interprets as Martín addresses me.

"I didn't think you were really handicapped until the lights came up. When I saw that you really were, my heart sort of stopped for a second. I was amazed. You expressed how I feel. I really feel like you are my brother. I feel like we have a strong connection. From heart to heart."

This is it.

Not something else.

This.

Thank you, Martín.

~

It's August now, and I'm back in Berkeley, between engagements. I just got a call from Sandy Gleysteen at *The Sunday Today Show* at NBC. They're sending out a crew to film me for three days. Maria Shriver is going to do the interview. National television. Coast to coast. Six million viewers. I can't believe it.

Right away, I sit down and write a letter to Sandy:

Dear Sandy,

I know that there is a great pull to make me look like a courageous human being who has fought so well against this deadly disease. I feel this pull, too. I recommend that you fight this pull and see me instead as a regular person living his own unique life. I recommend that the focus of the show be exploring what life is all about. I know you have deadlines to meet, but I hope you can take your time with me. Please consider staying in my apartment while you're here. There is space on my floor and I have an extra futon. Uncovering reality takes time.

Sincerely,
Neil Marcus

I read in *Newsweek* that just before the Presidential Debates earlier this month, Vice President Bush was nervous, so his advisor told him, "You just go out there and have fun." Bush glared at him and snapped, "You go out there and have fun in front of five million people!"

I get it, Mr. Bush.

Three … Two … One. Live.

They film me at home, at Mark O'Brien's, on the street, in a store, talking to Daniel, walking with Roger, eating in a cafeteria, interacting with a group of friends.

Then they film the interview with Maria Shriver at my apartment. She tells me she got a kick out of my invitation to her producer, Sandy.

I tell her that I'd never seen anybody like myself on TV before.

She says she hasn't either. She says, "We're breaking new ground here, Neil."

My cranky neighbor wanders in through my front door, past the crew, and into the shot. "What's going on here?" he says, cameras rolling. "What are you up to now?" He eyes everyone with suspicion, especially me. "I don't know about you, Marcus. I'm watching you." The crew just smiles and waits him out.

Then, it's over, and I go to my sister Kendra's house in the hills behind Berkeley and collapse.

And so, on September 11, 1988, the front room of my apartment is packed with friends and neighbors watching as the host, Garrick Utley, presents the news of the day. Texas is still reeling from Hurricane Gilbert. Then—

> GARRICK UTLEY: This morning on Sunday Today, we want to look at and listen to those among us for whom each day is a particularly difficult one in a way that most of us cannot even imagine. They are the disabled. It is time now to talk about being disabled, or rather listen to them, those who through disease or accident

cannot do what most of us take for granted: speaking, hearing, controlling our bodies.

MARIA SHRIVER: Neil Marcus spent an idyllic childhood playing with his four older brothers and sisters. But his world changed suddenly and drastically when, at the age of eight, he became afflicted with a rare neurological disorder called dystonia. Today, he is an award-winning playwright and actor. Neil, how does it make you feel when you go out there on that stage and perform your own words and tell people how you feel?

NEIL MARCUS: It feels good. I'm out there with everything I've got.

MARIA SHRIVER: What motivated you to create this play and to perform it?

NEIL MARCUS: Disabled people need more exposure out in the world.

MARIA SHRIVER: What is the message you're trying to convey?

NEIL MARCUS: I understand that the world wants you to believe you're insignificant.

MARIA SHRIVER: And you know you're not.

NEIL MARCUS: Yes.

MARIA SHRIVER: That's a big victory.

NEIL MARCUS: I think it's the biggest victory.

～

My words are simple, but important. I am answering the invitation to join *The Incredible Shrinking Man,* to step into the subatomic mist. I am echoing Cyrano: "No, thank you!" I am a gladiator slaying invisibility.

I have a few quibbles with the way they described me, but at least Maria Shriver had the wisdom not to pat me on the head.

After the show we have a very loud party. I even invite my cranky neighbor. He's a no-show.

～

It's late December. The play has been booked solid ever since *The Today Show* piece. And today I learned that *Storm Reading* will have two performances in Ford's Theatre in Washington, D.C., I am thrilled!

I'm also scared stiff.

39
AN EAST COAST THING
The Door to the Big Time Opens

May 1989
The best-selling non-fiction book is *A Brief History of Time*.
A million protestors swarm into Tiananmen Square in Beijing.

~

LAST WEEKEND, I WENT to the UC Santa Barbara campus to hear Stephen Hawking's lecture on baby black holes. This man is the latest model to come off nature's evolutionary assembly line. He can't walk. He uses an electric wheelchair and fixes his eyes on words on a computer screen to talk. He has expanded humanity's understanding of the universe more than anyone since Albert Einstein.

~

I'm on the bed in my apartment in Santa Barbara, reading a script.

I still have my place in Berkeley, but I've been staying here during the breaks between tours, because this is where the cast and crew are. Posters and paintings I've picked up while on tour are on the walls. A copy of the poster from our Denver performance is on the end of the bed. The room is a mess. The cable TV doesn't work.

The script I'm reading includes only three scenes from the play. That's because after the two Ford's Theatre engagements, we're going to perform these scenes in the Concert Hall of the Kennedy Center. It's part of a gala performance called *From the Heart*. It's the grand finale of the First International Very Special Arts Festival. Michael Douglas will introduce *Storm Reading*. He and I will exchange lines on stage. It doesn't seem quite real.

But that's not all. NBC is going to tape the gala performance and broadcast the whole thing as a network special. So. *Storm Reading* is going to be on national television. In prime time. Coast to coast. This is the big time. We have the opportunity to put a fresh, new, positive view of disability in the national spotlight. We're ready to do our bit.

There's a knock at the door.

"Come. In."

A guy in khaki carries in two blue buckets of tools and wires and stuff. His name patch says, "Sean." He's about my age, with a long blonde ponytail and a baseball cap.

"I'm here to fix your cable," says Sean. "Is this a good time?" he asks, glancing around.

"Sure."

"It'll probably just take a minute." Sean pulls the dresser forward and starts plugging and unplugging cable box connections, studying a small metal gadget. Then he notices the poster on the end of the bed. "That's you, right? So, you're the star of the show?" He seems pleased.

"Yeah."

Sean stops fiddling with the box. He looks at me. He sees me. He says, "I'm not really doing all the things that I want to do. But I can see that you are."

"Yes. I. Am." I'd like to say a lot more to him, but this will have to do.

"Good for you."

I look at him.

He means it. "I used to work for the cable company. Now I'm a free-lance eco-warrior, helping the little guy against the big corporations." Sean is smiling.

"Sean. We. All. Do. What. We. Can. Yeah?"

He looks surprised, and even more pleased.

"That we do. That we do." Sean's smile is wide now.

As Sean strips some coaxial cable, I try to imagine how this brief exchange might affect his worldview. The phone rings.

Sean says, "You want me to get it for you?"

"No. I. Got. It."

He hands me the phone.

"Hi, Neil. How are you? Getting some well-deserved rest, I hope." It's Rod.

"I'm good."

"Neil? I'm going to need your Social Security Number. Do you have that with you?" There's a playful lilt in his voice.

"No, I don't." It's at home in Berkeley.

"Well, could you get that number to me right away?"

"Yes. Why?" It would just take a call to Ojai. My parents have a copy.

"Well, Neil. Without your Social Security Number, they won't let you in the White House."

I am speechless.

Rod reads, "President George Herbert Walker Bush requests the presence of Neil Marcus at the White House for a Reception to Honor the Participants in The First International Very Special Arts Festival."

"I'll. Get. It. Now!" is all I can say.

"Okay," says Rod, "call me soon."

Looking up, I realize that Sean has overheard the whole conversation. He is standing there with his arms hanging loosely at his sides, his eyes wide, his mouth part-way open.

Then Sean says just one short word. It was the way that he said the word that impressed me, not the word itself. The overtones surrounding his voice were like those one might hear from the bystanders in a torch-lit tomb when a dust-covered sarcophagus lid is moved aside for the first time in thousands of years. There was a reverence as well, of the sort that is evoked only in the presence of the truly miraculous, like Michael Jackson moonwalking.

Sean whispered, "Dude."

My mom drives down from Ojai and takes me to the Catholic Charities Thrift Store in Santa Barbara to help me pick out a suit for the White House reception. An aproned salesperson with the name tag "Celia" approaches us as we are looking through the racks, "Are you looking for anything in particular?"

"He's been invited to the White House to meet the President," my mom says airily, as she double-checks the sleeve length on a light wool suit. Celia goes to tell the other salespeople and soon everyone's gathered around. They're really excited. When my mom explains that it's a reception on the lawn at the White House, a flurry of activity is set off as people measure my arms and chest, while others pick out suits appropriate for Washington DC in the early summer. I settle on a light-weight beige suit.

Just before we went back on tour, a group of us had dinner and went to the premiere of *My Left Foot*. Daniel Day Lewis plays Christy Brown, an Irishman who wrote masterpieces with his toes. Cerebral palsy. A true story. But just as Dustin Hoffman isn't autistic, Daniel Day Lewis doesn't have CP. Neither of them is even disabled. Honestly? The part should have been mine.

I'm at the airport in Boston.

Without my wheelchair.

Our flight from Denver was delayed and my chair went on a different plane. We're in Terminal A and now they're telling us that we have to take the shuttle bus to Terminal C to get the chair. They don't have any way to get me to the shuttle bus. I don't usually go around in public without a chair. It's sort of like crawling and hopping combined. Okay, I can do this.

I work my way out the doors and over to where the bus stops, and, when it arrives, hop on and fall into a seat. The bus sits there, idling, with its doors open, and then two guys get on and sit to my left. Both of them are wearing Red Sox caps. The guy closest to me says, "Which terminal is this?" People don't usually ask me things like that. An autograph, sure, but directions? Rarely.

I say, "A."

The guy squints a little and says, "A?" Like he's not sure what I said.

So, as clearly as I can, I repeat, "A."

He pauses, then says, "A," not as a question really, but rising in pitch.

Then it occurs to me that he may be Canadian. I've heard Canadians say "eh" a lot. So I just say, "Yeah," not knowing what else to say.

He turns away, looking a little confused. The bus starts up. We're swaying around a bit. The guy is talking to his friend, on the other side of him. We sway some more. Then the friend leans around and, pointing at the guy, says, "He thought you were Canadian. Because you said 'eh.' They always say 'eh.' You know what I mean?" He gives a one-burst laugh.

Then I say, "I. Am. Ca. Na. Dian."

They get it. We all start laughing at once. I'm still smiling as the bus pulls up to Terminal C.

Two performances tomorrow in Cambridge. Then a series of one-night stands, three nights in Baltimore, winding our way down toward Washington and Ford's Theatre.

We've performed *Storm Reading* dozens of times now, in front of thousands of people. Based on audience responses, we've adjusted some of the timing and rewritten several scenes. It's a much better play now. More finely tuned. It's ready.

And the doubts and fears that I had when we started out are much smaller now. The treatment that has shrunk them is applause, glowing reviews, standing ovations, and thousands of words of thanks and encouragement from enthusiastic fans. And, of course, hours of practice. I'm ready.

I know that some people see me as a token. I get that, and they're not entirely wrong, but I'm on the stage now, under the lights, and I'm going to seize the moment.

Every serious artist dreams of creating a work that moves people, that stirs them up inside, that makes them rattle their cages, that makes them scream and yell and laugh and cry. They also want that work to widen people's vision and sharpen their perception of reality. I've done that. People come up to me all the time and tell me that I have changed the way they see the world. After one performance, a boy with what looked like cerebral palsy came up to me and said, "Your. Play. Made. Me. Proud. To. Be. Spastic!"

And now, the audience for this work will be measured in the millions.

I'm ready.

I roll out onto the stage in Cambridge. It's the middle of the play. In the audience are some people in motorized beds. My fans, a whole nation of people eager to join in the game of life, people who have been benched. I pause center stage, facing left. There is a rope, taut now, angling upward from my chair to the shadows in the wings behind me.

The theater is silent. I abruptly push the joystick all the way forward. As the chair lurches forward, a suitcase is yanked from the shadows and falls about eight feet, crashing to the stage with a loud *thunk*. I drag it off, stage left.

My letter to Samsonite luggage is projected on the big screen at the back of the stage. Roger reads it. Kathryn translates it into sign language.

Dear Samsonite,

I love your ads. The football team tackling your hard-shell luggage. The karate master attacking a pile of your carry-ons. The gorilla beating up a leather tote.

I have always wanted to see you do an ad where a person in a wheelchair is doing something really brutal with one of your suitcases.

People tend to fear that if you bring disability into public view, you are making fun of the people who have disabilities in a way that is rude. I don't think this is the case.

Please consider using disabled people in your ads.

Sincerely,
Neil Marcus

It's good schtick, and a serious call for people to wake up. The audience loves it.

Next stop: Washington, D.C.

40
A Date With Fate

In the National Arena

June 12, 1989

In March, *Rain Man* won Best Picture.

On June 3, the People's Liberation Army killed thousands of students in Tiananmen Square.

The next day, a man carrying his shopping bags stood his ground in front of a PLA tank.

~

I'M ON THE FLAT ROOF of the Kennedy Center in Washington, D.C.

Above me, all around me, are giant, dark clouds, low and churning. I'm standing, leaning on my chair. Bursts of wind blast me in the face, then push me from behind. Powerful gusts. I stumble, almost lose my balance. A seemingly opaque storm cloud, just there, over the river, is suddenly lit from within by an exchange of lightning bolts that flash, but never strike the earth. Then thunder, so low and loud that my bones vibrate.

Right now, I am Spartacus, arriving in chains in the capital of my imperial masters, surrounded by majestic columned edifices clad in marble that echo the pride and grandeur of ancient Rome. Soon, I shall wrap my chains around these columns and pull them down. I, Spartacus, shall prevail against the might of Rome.

Suddenly, a waterfall of rain. All at once. I rush to the stairwell, pull open the metal door and hurry inside. Too late. I am drenched.

This tempest was a herald, announcing the arrival of *Storm Reading* to the capital. Maybe.

∾

When I was little, and I became disabled, I didn't really know what "disabled" meant. I simply knew it was something that was not good. I also knew it was something to be greatly feared. But how did I know these things?

The knowledge must have seeped into my consciousness from the language used around me. I heard about people who were "victims" of polio, or "suffered" from cerebral palsy, or were "afflicted" by "mental retardation." People in car accidents were "threatened" with paralysis. It was always said that wheelchairs were something you "succumbed" to. And, of course, people were "confined" to a wheelchair. All the words and images associated with disability were filled with dread, gloom, and doom. I learned that it was horrible to be the "cripple." I learned harsh lessons from *Heidi*.

While still in my teens, I looked around and saw how few of the images of disability were positive. I decided that this negative image of disability needed changing. After all, I was still disabled and was probably going to continue being disabled, and I wanted to enjoy my life and my future. I also wanted people with disabilities to feel proud, to feel like they belonged.

I guess I sort of stumbled upon art as the best tool for the job. And people responded very positively. If a disability culture could take root, and be nurtured, then it could grow into a thing of beauty.

For the next two nights, *Storm Reading* will be on the stage at Ford's Theatre. This weekend, it will take the stage at the Kennedy Center Concert Hall. In the annals of disability culture, this will be a groundbreaking event. There has never been anything like it.

〜

Ford's Theatre. I make my entrance, unseen. Then I rise up from the darkness silhouetted by bright swirling colors. I'm out there on stage for the next 90 minutes. I am like a prize fighter, stretching the limits of my endurance, using every corner of the ring. In constant motion, like Muhammed Ali. Sweating. Pouring sweat. Going to the wings for water between the acts. To get the sweat mopped off. I follow all the traffic patterns of the script, zig-zagging back and forth across the stage right on cue. Now I'm at Burger King. Now I'm a movie star. Now I'm in an opera. In a rainforest. A hospital. A park. Now I'm at home in bed. I'm being knighted by kings and queens and then beings from a parallel universe. I'm everywhere.

You have to experience it to understand how it feels to have the energy of life flow through you, with the channel wide open.

〜

During the curtain call at the end of our second night, I look out at the standing, clapping, cheering audience, then over at the empty box seat, where Abraham Lincoln was shot. I know it sounds funny, immodest even, but, in a way, *Storm Reading* is like the Emancipation Proclamation. I'm not kidding.

The spastic emerges, is seen. He tells a joke, then stands tall. He asks for indulgence, risks his life, then declares his freedom, and takes a bow. I think Lincoln might approve. This play liberates people.

〜

Roger and I are interviewed by Linda Wertheimer for National Public Radio's *All Things Considered* the following day. Afterward, Rod tells me that this one interview is likely to generate more interest in *Storm Reading* than all the other radio interviews we've done put together.

In a few days, I'm going to the White House.

41
STORMING THE WHITE HOUSE
A Spastic on the South Lawn

June 1989

Yesterday, Ronald Reagan was knighted by Queen Elizabeth II.

THE GUARD AT THE visitors' entrance to the White House is stumped. His job today was supposed to be straightforward. There is a reception on the South Lawn for the Very Special Arts Festival. He has the guest list on his clipboard. When a guest comes up to his guardhouse, all he has to do is compare the identification provided by the guest with the information on the list, and, if they match, check off the guest's name, provide the embossed name tag, and welcome the guest to the reception.

Except.

In front of him is a man with no identification. The guard works his jaw. No driver's license. No passport. Two clean-shaven bumps rise and fall, one below each ear. Not even a credit card.

The security protocols are crystal clear. No one is allowed to enter the White House grounds who has not been properly cleared. These protocols are not mere formalities. They are designed to protect the life of the President of the United States of America, George Herbert Walker Bush. The eyes of the guard narrow and harden as he prepares to launch into his carefully rehearsed "I'm very sorry, sir, but without proper identification" speech.

But he hesitates.

He hesitates because many of the guests today have disabilities and this man with no papers is in a wheelchair. So, there's that.

Then there's the fact that this man seems to be only marginally in control of his movements and speech. While it is conceivable that this is the clever ruse of a would-be assassin bent on revenge against the House of Bush, the guard suspects that it is not. The friends of the unidentified spastic have all passed muster. Their identification matches the information on the list. Check, check, and check. And they all swear that their friend is who he claims to be.

But. The rules are the rules. And the possibility exists, however remotely, that the frame of this wheelchair has been filled with explosives. And his job is to follow the rules, to prevent the unthinkable.

The guard clears his throat as I reach behind me. Slowly. No sudden movements. He pauses and watches me closely. I extract a cardboard tube from the pouch on the back of my chair. Roger catches on. He removes the rolled up poster from the tube and unrolls it. Again, slowly.

The poster announces that Neil Marcus will be performing his play, *Storm Reading*, at Ford's Theatre on Monday and Tuesday. From the poster, my picture smiles up at the guard. Utilizing all that I have learned about theater after a grueling year on the road, I duplicate that smile and turn to face the guard.

He smiles back, checks my name off the guest list, and hands me my embossed name-tag.

～

The crowd is clustered on one side of the pavilion on the South Lawn and, as we approach, people step aside, creating a path between me and the center of the cluster. When I get to the front, there's the President, on a small stage, telling us how great we are. When he finishes his speech, balloons are released. There's a lot of jostling. People standing around me. I can't see very well. I'm sort of pushed further to the front and then, here I am, face to face with the man himself, President Bush. And the First Lady, Barbara Bush.

The President of the United States offers me his right hand. I take it with my left and shake it. I look him in the eye. And then he sees me. I can tell. He is not seeing an inspiring handicapped playwright or a brave victim who overcame his disability. He sees me, here in front of him. Not a soap opera, a Disney yarn, or a made-for-TV movie. He is shaking my hand and we connect. Man to man. He seems to be a little startled by it. Then he smiles. I smile back and say, "Hello."

42

BEING GREEN

Starstruck and Dazzled

Friday, June 17, 1989
The Solidarity Party is elected in Poland.
The #1 Song is "Wind Beneath My Wings," sung by Bette Midler.

~

I'M IN THE GREEN ROOM at the Kennedy Center Concert Hall, waiting to be called to the stage. The performance tonight will be taped for broadcast as *From the Heart*, an NBC special featuring many of the artists from the First International Very Special Arts Festival, and lots of other celebrities. So, while there are only 3,500 people in the audience tonight, they say that in September there will be a television audience of more than six million.

The green room is off to the side of the stage and down a short flight of stairs. Because there's no elevator or ramp, I had to get here by hopping down the stairs. The festival artists who use wheelchairs and can't hop aren't here. They're waiting off-stage somewhere else. There's no law saying that theaters must make their green rooms accessible to wheelchairs. I've had to wrestle my way up and down stairs in many of the places that have hosted

Storm Reading. And lots of those stairs didn't even have handrails. But still, the Kennedy Center?

I met Tony Melendez, a singer who plays his guitar with his feet because he has no arms. He told me that the broadcast version of the show will include a clip of him performing for Pope John Paul II in Los Angeles. The Pope hugged and kissed him. More about hugs later.

When it was time for me to go on stage to rehearse yesterday, Rich, my attendant, abruptly picked me up and carried me up onto the stage like I was a baby. I was mortified and angry. To be fair, all the surrounding glitz and glamor may have momentarily befuddled him. I knew better than to let it distract me from my performance. He should have known better, though. And there should have been a ramp.

During rehearsal we did the "Burger King" scene from the play. Then NBC told us that they had called Burger King while we were rehearsing. Burger King wouldn't give us permission to use its name or sing its song on national television. So tonight, it will be "Burger Boy." If you ask me, I think Burger King let a golden opportunity for free publicity slip right through its greasy fingers.

Today, while I was waiting to have my makeup done, in the chair ahead of me was Ellen Burstyn. A few years ago, I saw her in the movie *Resurrection*. She played Edna, a woman with the power to heal. In one scene, she places her hands on a girl named Louise who has dystonia. Somehow, all of the symptoms are passed over from Louise to Edna. Ellen Burstyn did a great job in the scene. I was so impressed. I really felt like I had a bond with her. When she was done with makeup, she got up from her chair, and turned toward me. In my enthusiasm, I blurted out, "Hi, Ellen!"

This is how you learn that simply because you feel a special bond with a celebrity, it does not necessarily follow that the celebrity in question feels a special bond with you. I felt like such a dork. Like I had on a white football helmet.

About an hour later, Kenny Rogers walked by me and casually said, "Hi, Neil."

I know it's not the same thing, but still, I mean, I was shocked. I felt like Nelson Rockefeller.

Terry Angus just left to go on stage. When he was 17, he made his own Kermit the Frog puppet, shot a video, and sent it to Jim Henson, asking for an audition. He has been working with the Muppets ever since. Right now, he's on stage with Jim Henson. Kermit the Frog is singing a duet with Terry's Fake Kermit. They're singing "It Isn't Easy Being Green." Terry has cerebral palsy. Which isn't so easy, either. It could be that what originally drew Terry to puppetry was that the puppeteer is hidden. If that's right, his cunning plan backfired. Pretty soon, more than six million people will watch Jim Henson walk across the stage with Terry. You can't really hide, anyway. When I met Kermit, I got tongue-tied. Star-struck, I guess.

Kathryn just told me that we're up next. Got to go.

43

SHOWDOWN AT THE OK CORRAL

A Line of Respect Is Drawn

June 17, 1989, continued

❧

NIGHT.

I'm back at the hotel. It's late. I can't sleep. I'm looking out the window at the Watergate complex across the street. It's raining now.

Sometimes, acting feels a lot like brain surgery. The bright lights. The air, heavy with tension. The drenching sweat. The pressure. And the relief when it's over.

I'm going over the performance in my mind.

❧

First, Michael Douglas, alone on the stage, explains that *Storm Reading*, unlike most plays, has the dimension of "absolute truth," because it is an autobiographical play, performed by the playwright.

Exactly.

He is telling them that this is not make-believe. Then I roll out from stage left, and hand him my diary, from which he will read excerpts between the three abbreviated scenes.

I launch into the opening. "People are watching me. People are watching me all the time …" While my torso, and especially my leg, are fully involved tonight, my speech is quite clear. This is good. Kathryn comes out, then Roger. After Roger says his last line, Michael Douglas reads from the diary about my determination that "the show must go on," regardless of how I feel on any particular night. So far, so good.

The second scene is "Burger Boy." The audience eats it up. Then Michael Douglas reads from my diary, about my anxiety before one performance, my confidence before another. I'm like a lion. Let me at 'em!" Everything is working.

For the third and final scene, Roger speaks while a camera focuses on my face, close up.

"I believe I have a voice. Words, feelings, observations, perceptions, thoughts that can move the world. I am a storm, a cyclone of ideas, thunder and lightning, a warm summer's breeze, a gentle spring rain."

Knowing that the close-ups of my head will be larger than life on millions of TV screens makes me feel self-conscious. I do my best to have the position of my head, my facial expression, and my eyes convey the meaning, the feeling of the words as they are spoken. The tension of dystonia in my face adds to the power of the expression. It works.

"Some people hide from storms. They close their shutters and doors and blinds. They steep themselves in their own darkness and rob themselves of the tumultuous journey and its exhilaration."

I squint, close my eyes, and turn my head. Expressing willful withdrawal.

"Some people, when they see my twisted frame, my dystonic disarray, embrace the storm. Their eyes light up and they rush to hug me as a long lost brother. As if embracing a storm was food for their soul."

As Kathryn embraces me to translate these words, I look at her directly and express their warmth, and affection.

"I can teach you … to read a storm."

At this, I hold my face at rest, relaxed, conveying quiet confidence with my eyes, as they scan the audience. Then Michael Douglas walks over to shake my hand, and we exit, stage left.

There's a story behind that handshake.

I watch the rest of the show from the wings. The last act is Melissa Manchester singing "Over the Rainbow." As she is belting out her final "why can't I," Lauren Bacall walks over to me, leans over, and says, "Just stick with me. This is for you."

And so, for the grand finale, I escort Lauren Bacall to the stage, in Humphrey Bogart's place. She stands by my side as the entire cast comes on stage. Together, we sing the final verse of "Over the Rainbow." The lyrics are Yip Harburg's. He was blacklisted in the 1950s, for dreaming of better land. "Why, oh why, can't I?"

Amazing.

~

Now about that handshake.

During rehearsal, as I was handing Michael Douglas my diary, the director told him to give me a hug.

Well.

As soon as this direction was given, Rod, who had been watching from the fifth row, rose from his seat, walked down the aisle to the stage and asked to have a word with the director.

In principle, I have nothing against hugs. In fact, you could say that, if battle lines were being drawn, I would be in the "pro-hug" camp. Generally speaking, I believe that our society would benefit from more human contact. But we are not speaking generally here.

Imagine for a moment that Michael Douglas is seated, center stage, at the start of a performance of his successful autobiographical play, in which he stars as himself. Now imagine that he hands his play diary to Senator Edward M. Kennedy, who is standing next to him. Then imagine Senator Kennedy leaning over and giving Mr. Douglas a nice big hug.

Which is to say that context matters.

Although hugging between adult males has lost some of its stigma in America, this imagined scenario demonstrates that it is not yet gone. How could you change the scenario to make the embrace seem less awkward?

If they were both standing, that would help. Or if they were brothers, or cousins, somehow related, that could help, too. Even if they were just old friends who had worked together for years, who had formed a lasting bond, that would probably be enough to nudge the hug out of the column labeled "inappropriate." But the surest way to make Ted Kennedy hugging a seated Michael Douglas seem appropriate would be to magically transform the latter into a three-year-old. Into little Mikey Douglas.

To be clear, then. Michael Douglas and I were not both standing. We are not relatives. We are not old chums.

And I am not three years old.

From the edge of the stage, Rod addressed the director. "Couldn't you just have Mr. Douglas and Mr. Marcus shake hands?"

"What? You mean, lose the hug?" asked the director, wrinkling his brow.

"It's just that I think Mr. Marcus prefers handshakes," said Rod, hoping for a swift and just settlement.

"But the hug works. If we lose the hug, it doesn't work. It's got no heart." His tone was plaintive. The hope for a quick resolution was fading.

Then Rod, ever the interpersonal tactician, called in reinforcements. "What do you think, Neil?"

"Hand. Shake," I said. I was not a toddler.

Still addressing Rod, the director said, "I'm telling you, the audience will love the hug. It works."

Rod: "Neil?" Strongly suggesting that the decision was mine to make. Good move.

I fixed my gaze on the director. "No. Hug."

As I watched, the director looked over at Rod and carefully considered his next move.

I don't know what went on in his head but, whatever it was, it took him less than two seconds. And from his look, I could tell that, in the case of Hug v. Handshake, Hug had prevailed.

Then he turned and looked at me. And I think he saw in my eyes something similar to what I had detected in the set of the jaw of Blind Chuck. I think he saw that I was unlikely to change my opinion, hugwise. I think he saw that the bearded man in the wheelchair in front of him was not going to be infantilized. It is also possible he noticed that Mr. Marcus was not a toddler. Maybe.

Still looking at me, he turned his attention to things that really matter. "You okay with a handshake, Mr. Douglas?"

"Not a problem with me. But why don't we put the handshake at the end?" Michael Douglas suggested.

"Perfect," said the director, without satisfaction, and we were past the rapids.

In 1973, Marlon Brando won the Oscar for Best Actor. At the ceremony, Sacheen Little Feather, speaking on his behalf, explained that Mr. Brando was refusing the award to protest the portrayal of Native Americans by the film industry. As she was speaking, members of the American Indian Movement, including Dennis Banks, were occupying the town of Wounded Knee, South Dakota.

I am not comparing myself to Marlon Brando. All I'm saying is that he inspired me to stand my ground. He gave me courage.

Thank you, Mr. Brando. And thank you, Mr. Douglas.

44
HEART STRINGS ATTACHED
Enigmas of Human Motivation

June 17, 1989, continued

~

NIGHT.

From the window of my dark hotel room, I watch streetlights dance on wet pavement. Dawn soon. I've got to get some sleep. But I can't stop thinking about something I saw during the dress rehearsal.

~

Seated in the middle of the tenth row, watching the rehearsal, I am thinking about Very Special Arts, the foundation that is sponsoring the event. It was founded by Jean Kennedy Smith. She's the younger sister of one president and two senators. I think of JFK. I remember his rocking chair, PT 109, and the album that spoofed *Camelot, The First Family*. I think of his father, Joe, Sr., sipping his drink on the porch in Hyannis Port.

As the hostess for the evening, Jean will speak from the stage, as will her brother Teddy, and his son, Ted, Jr., both of whom are seated in the row right in front of me. And this stage itself is, of course, in the Kennedy Center. In a way, the Kennedys are like American royalty. It occurs to me that this show will be as close as we come in America to a command performance. Tomorrow night, the Kennedys will be joined by the Bushes. I am struck by the dazzling fame, the vast fortunes, and the awesome power that will fill this hall.

And everyone will be here to help create opportunities in the arts for people with disabilities. So noble, so selfless. It's wonderful.

In one of the first numbers, Gary Morris, who sang in *Les Miserables*, is joined on stage by dozens of young people with disabilities, most of them singing along with him. As he winds up, he kneels next to a little girl, then picks her up, so that she's seated on his forearm. As the music moves up a half-step, the harp signaling the key change, the little girl puts her index finger in her mouth and sucks on it, looking out at the audience with wide eyes. Gary doesn't miss a beat. At the end, he hits a high C and holds it. Very moving.

In the next number, as Kenny Rogers, who won a Grammy for "The Gambler," sings another inspiring ballad, a huge screen behind him shows footage shot the day before at the White House. The music is slow, building, filled with violins. On the screen, a blind boy, about ten years old, is singing with Kenny on the South Lawn stage. He may be Filipino. Together, they sing, "When you put your heart in it, it can take you anywhere," then there's a long pause.

The boy says, "Mr. President George Bush, may I shake your hand? I would like to know how different the hand of a president is from a blind boy like me. Okay?"

This makes me feel, I don't know, sad, maybe. Then, with the violins still playing, George Bush, five times life size, leaves his front row seat on the White House lawn, bounds up the steps to the stage, shakes the boy's hand, wraps his other arm around him, then pulls him close and kisses the top of his head. All on this huge screen. The sadness, or whatever it is, is growing stronger now. I'm getting a lump in my throat, tears in my eyes. The President delivers a few words from the podium, then, on a wave of violins, with the chorus sounding like so many angels, Kenny winds it up.

> Suddenly it happens.
> A chance in a lifetime.
> Now we're gonna take it.
> We can make it.
> When you put your heart in it.

~

And then, *pop!*

The noble and selfless enterprise in front of me disappears. Oh, nothing has changed. It is the same music, the same performers, the same narration. But it is no longer a performance with the sole purpose of creating opportunities in the arts for people with disabilities. That performance has been transformed into a very different show.

I didn't ask to see this. I didn't really want to see this. But I see it. Let me try to explain.

Look at the little blind kid walking off stage with the star who just hugged him. Now, listen to the fanfare. That music is designed to make you cry, isn't it? The violins, the crescendos, they put a lump in your throat. Don't they? Go ahead the music says, let it all out. Go ahead, cry. Express your pity.

Or look at the girl whose head is inches from the singer's mouth as he hits that high note. She is deaf. She can't hear him. Who is he singing to?

It is allowed to look at disability here. That's the idea. It's a show. The usual rules about ogling at disability don't apply. Not here, not now. Go ahead. Stare.

And that celebrity wouldn't be up there if there were something inappropriate about hugging a singing blind kid, would he? Or singing to a deaf girl? Of course not. This show is sanctioned. You can indulge your fearful curiosity about disability, the desire to look that you feel alongside that desire to look away, and not feel pangs of guilt. Go ahead. Gawk.

P.T. Barnum showcased Tom Thumb and the Bearded Lady, and Cheng and Eng, the original Siamese Twins. But that was different; that was exploitation without pity. Straight up heartless reveling in the fascination of human difference for fun, and for profit, too. This show, on the other hand, is about doing good. And yet, somehow, right now, it seems to me that Mr. Barnum would probably feel right at home sitting in the seat next to me.

The founder of Very Special Arts is addressing the audience now. Her older sister was born with cognitive and neurological disabilities. She was lobotomized and placed in an "institution" about 48 years ago. She's still in there. I ask myself how the Very Special Arts Foundation fits into that ethical puzzle. I'm not sure.

Consider that Washington power broker who feels that life has been very good, but feels a twinge of guilt about those to whom life has not been so good? This is a chance to open his checkbook and give. It will make him look good, he'll probably feel better, and the donation will probably help some people with disabilities, but at what cost?

An unpleasant question poses itself. Is this charity in part a device employed by the powerful to assuage their feelings of guilt? Is it a ritual held to numb the pain of inequity and injustice? Is it a ceremony of atonement for callous acts that may have seemed so necessary on the ascent to wealth and power? Is this show a "good work" put on to gain an indulgence?

To be blunt: who is really meant to benefit from this charitable event? Who is it really for?

There are people who have mastered the skill of not facing unpleasant truths. My life experience has rendered me relatively incapable of self-deception. I find it hard to fool myself.

Seated here in the middle of the tenth row, I am now facing an uninvited, unwanted truth. I have the sense that I am seeing the back of something that most people see only the front of. This event is, at least in part, a festival of sanctioned pity, soothed guilt, self-promotion, and morbid curiosity.

That's how it looks from the middle of the tenth row, anyway.

❧

Then, *pop!* The noble, selfless gala performance reappears. In an eyeblink. The dark show is gone, the bright show is back.

I am both grateful and proud that *Storm Reading* was part of *From the Heart*. I really am. But human motives are almost never pure. Every complex human undertaking is propelled by a mixture of motives. It would be childish to think otherwise. And I hope that by now we've established that I'm not a child.

The people who put together *From the Heart* were motivated by a sense of fairness, generosity, kindness, and respect. I don't doubt this. But in this mix of people and motives, I also discern shadows of guilt, greed, pity, exploitation and self-aggrandizement. I take no pleasure in pointing it out. But I can't unsee something once I've seen it.

I can imagine a different production. One that doesn't spend so much time jerking tears, tugging heartstrings, and kissing and hugging little kids with disabilities.

❧

The rain has stopped. I am staring now not out the window but in it, at my reflection.

What are you going to do now, Mr. Marcus? You're 35 years old.

How can you possibly top that?

45
WHAT IS MY ROLE?
Opportunity Knocking

September 1993
The Cold War is over.
***The X-Files* premiered last week.**

∽

STORM READING IS ON hiatus. I'm going to rest here in Berkeley and catch up with friends. My sister Wendy isn't working, so she's moved down from her place in Northern California and into my spare bedroom. She's eight years older than me and a wonderful cook. She's eager to help and having her here makes things easier for me.

Since being showcased on *From the Heart*, we've performed for 200 live audiences in more than 30 states. I can say my lines in my sleep. Roger is leaving the show, handing his part to Matthew Ingersoll.

A film crew toured with us for a while, shooting a documentary about Access Theatre called *Speaking Through Walls*. Anthony Edwards, who played Goose in *Top Gun*, directed. He's from Santa Barbara and has worked with Rod on several projects.

In Vancouver, at a performance sponsored by the founders of the Dystonia Medical Research Foundation, we put on *Storm Reading* for a house full of doctors. A few eyes were opened.

Last summer, I met Remy Charlip at a poetry reading. He's an accomplished artist and founding member of the Merce Cunningham Dance Company. We hit it off. I hope to explore dance with him, to learn as much as I can from him. He is a mentor and good friend.

Mark O'Brien has been pretty busy. He's been selling poems, and *The Sun* published his autobiographical essay, "On Seeing a Sex Surrogate." I introduced him to Jessica Yu, who wants to make a documentary film about his life.

Yesterday, I was being interviewed about disability culture here at home by a friend who just got a fellowship from the National Rehabilitation Institute when the phone rang. The answering machine picked up.

"Hi, Neil, this is Rod. If you're there, would you please pick up?"

I pick up. "Hi."

"Neil, CBS just called. They've offered you a part in a TV pilot called *Christy*."

My mind raced. *Christy*? Oh, my god! This is the TV sequel to *My Left Foot*, the biography of Christy Brown! Daniel Day Lewis probably told CBS, "No. Been there, done that. It's Neil's turn now!"

I've finally made it to the top! This is it! I'm going to play Christy Brown!

Rod put the producer on the line. He tells us that *Christy* is about a young woman in the early 1900s who leaves the city to teach in a small community, where she learns a lot about herself and about life, especially from a character named Wilmer who is a sort of "wild man." Oh.

Tyne Daley will play a leader of the community. The pilot will be filmed in the Great Smoky Mountains. The part being offered is, of course, Wilmer, the "wild man." He is the son of the poorest family in the community. At night, he sleeps in a cage. Ah.

In the beginning, Christy, the young teacher, is afraid of Wilmer who is "rambunctious in his physicality." He mentions frothing at the mouth. Thrashing around. Okay.

To the everlasting credit of the producers of this show, they want the part to be played by a real live disabled person. Face it, they could have called Richard Thomas who played John-Boy in *The Waltons*. Or any one of a hundred other abled actors.

Daniel says Wilmer is like a black "mammy" role in early cinema. Someone recently told me that the legendary Paul Robeson once said, "I'll do whatever it takes to get my black face up on that screen." Even actors like Lincoln Perry, who made millions playing the trickster Stepin Fetchit, did their part to blaze a trail for the Black actors who came after.

Well, I would like to get this twisted frame up on that screen. As I've said, I'll play any part offered until it is considered perfectly normal to see an actor who actually has a disability on screen.

"I'll. Do. It," I said. And, as rarely happens, I said it quite clearly on the first try.

The producer said, "Great! I'll get back to you with confirmation!"

I thought it was a done deal. "Okay. Thank. You."

Rod thanked him as well. After the producer hung up, Rod gave a small shriek.

46
GETTING THERE

Solo Cross-Country to the Shoot

October 1993

Last week, the Russian Army stormed the parliament building in Moscow. *What's Eating Gilbert Grape?* **is shooting on location in Pflugerville, Texas.**

I GOT THE PART!

They ask me for my shoe, shirt, waist, and inseam sizes, as well as my social security number. Done. I get strict instructions not to shave, not to trim my fingernails, and, more generally, not to groom myself for the duration. I can do that. They say that Rod and I will fly in on Sunday, shoot the scene with Christy on Monday, then fly home on Tuesday. Like a commando raid.

At least one of the producers of *Christy* seems to be having doubts that I am right for the part of Wilmer. Apparently, he convinced the others that Rod and I should kick in at least part of the air fare. It's not a big deal. With all the touring, I have lots of frequent flyer miles. Still, I do not consider this to be a good omen.

I go to buy a roundtrip ticket to Knoxville. I put my frequent flyer coupons on the counter. The transaction is complex, and I get flustered. My leg flies up, my head goes down, my torso twists to the left, and my speech gets all jammed up. A lively exchange with much misunderstanding ensues.

"Did you say 'Nashville?'"

"No. *Knox*. Ville." And on and on. The poor ticket agent thinks I'm having a seizure. He's so eager to help me on my way that he accepts the frequent flyer coupons without checking the expiration dates. My flight is in one week.

My seat is 38F, the very last row. The flight attendant graciously offers to help me get to my seat with an aisle chair, a narrow, purpose-built wheelchair. I even more graciously decline her offer and hop the length of the plane. At Aisle 38, I execute a complex maneuver that combines a pirouette with the characteristic squat step of a Cossack dancer. This lands me in the aisle seat next to a surprised sixtyish man dressed in blue jeans and a flannel shirt. His blue eyes, set in a ruddy face, blink just once. He knows what to do.

"Hi. Name's Bob." He shakes my hand.

The landscape of his accent is flat, with no mountains on the horizon in any direction. The voice of the Great Plains.

"I'm. Neil."

The landscape of my accent is the topology of M.C. Escher, with water flowing uphill, with the foreground in the background. We immediately hit it off.

Looking at my boarding pass, Bob says, "Looks like they assigned us the same seat. Well, that's okay. I'll just sit here, if that's okay with you."

"I'm. Good. Thanks," I say as I fish around for the other half of my seatbelt.

The gracious flight attendant appears and addresses me. "Sir? When you exit the plane may I suggest that you use the aisle chair instead of hobbling?"

I generously grant her permission to make the suggestion by saying, "Okay."

Hobbling? Really?

Then, showing thousands of dollars' worth of perfect teeth, she asks, "Do you need any help eating? Yes, or no?"

This is an intriguing proposal, but I think she lacks the good humor required to make it fun for everyone and therefore say, "No. I'll. Do. It."

I watch carefully but detect no trace of disappointment. As Bob helps me butter my muffin, he expresses confidence that his corn will be ready for harvest in less than a week. "The good Lord willing," he adds, unnecessarily.

In Chicago, Bob gets off and Rod gets on. In Knoxville, I race down the aisle behind the other passengers before help arrives. We're met by the director's assistant, who gets us settled in at our hotel and then drives us through the night to what he calls "the director's bunker." As we eat pizza, the director tells Rod and me about the script. Then he speaks directly to me.

"Frankly, Neil, I'm a little worried that some people will see you in a cage and think it's child abuse. But I'm savvy enough to make the scene so convincingly set in 1912 that the audience will see it as a realistic portrayal of the people of that time and place. That will deflect any criticism. Look, Neil, we didn't bring you here to evoke pity. My hope is that you can make the role of Wilmer shine. Understand?"

"Yes," I say, frankly.

"You'll be fine. No need to be nervous. Remember, we put our pants on one leg at a time, just like everyone else."

"That's. Right."

The phone rings. The director answers. As Rod and I sit there, the director talks with one of the producers about my scene, which is being shot tomorrow morning. It is clear that they don't know whether it will be shot indoors or out. They talk about more script changes. New lines. I get the impression that we're going to be doing improv, making it up as we go along.

47
ALKA-SELTZER

Acting in a Network Mini-Series

October 18, 1993

**The Dow Jones Industrial Average closes today at 3642. Trading is brisk.
Nelson Mandela and F.W. de Klerk are awarded the Nobel Peace Prize.**

⁓

THE NEXT MORNING WHEN we arrive at the set it's still dark out. There's this
whole compound in the mountains. Trailers, lights, security, generators. It
reminds me of the final set in *Close Encounters of the Third Kind*, at Devil's
Tower. Without thinking, I look up.

A golf cart takes me to makeup and wardrobe. My costume is a tattered
knee-length sweater that feels like burlap. My makeup is peanut butter
and oatmeal, carefully applied to simulate dirt, drool, grease, and snot. As
requested, I haven't shaved for a week, and am suitably stubbled. The same
makeup that is applied to my face, beard, and hair is also gently rubbed into
my teeth. Looking in the mirror, I see Wilmer.

In a clearing in the woods is a ramshackle old cabin, built by the crew
over the last week or so. This is the home of the O'Teales, Wilmer's family.

My family. It houses my mother, my two sisters, my two brothers, and the eldest child, me. I don't know where my father is. Outside the cabin there are chickens whose comportment is the concern of two chicken wranglers. Some of the chickens have been tethered to the earth with an invisible filament. They are indignant. Near the cabin are three fake rows of corn stalks. Two guys make sure the cabin is filled with smoke of just the right density. Apparently, it has been decided to shoot the scene indoors. The lighting crew makes the interior look just like early morning, which it is. The floor of the cabin is dirt. Next to a big table is my cage, with bars made from stout tree limbs. A pot of deer meat boils over a fire in the stone fireplace.

When we rehearse the scene, my sweater keeps falling off my shoulder so the sleeve gets all tangled up in my hand. It's very uncomfortable. I have to ask Rod to help me straighten it out. The director tells the costume guy, "Needs more holes. Needs more frayed edges." Our family is dirt poor. Rod has to help me again. As we rehearse the scene, over and over, Rod tries to direct me, signing, "Do this, do that." This is very hard to do in a small cabin with about twelve people crammed in the smoky morning gloom.

Suddenly, the makeup man comes over and sticks an Alka-Seltzer tablet into my mouth. It's so your mouth foams, I'm told. Boy, does it! My mouth fills with stinging foam. Around me, there's a mad rush. People are running around me in all directions.

"Quiet on the set! Wait. Get those footprints off the floor. Lose that reflection. Okay. Quiet! Roll 'em. Rolling. Aaaaand … action!"

Christy, the new teacher from the big city, is seated at a rough-hewn plank table across from my mother, Swannie O'Teale. They are discussing my little sister, Mountie, who has chosen not to talk. Christy is unaware that hiding under the table at her very feet, slathered in peanut butter and wearing a now truly tattered sweater, is me, Wilmer.

When Christy discovers me there, frothing at the mouth, she gasps. My mother notices and says, "Oh, that's Wilmer, my first born. Don't mind him. He's a good boy," and hands me a chunk of authentic 1900s cornbread. As I take a bite, she adds, "He was breech-born." At this, I become animated, eager to contribute to the discussion. Note: this will be my first speaking part on network television since *From the Heart.* I speak.

"Ah. Ahhhn. Ahhhh. Aahhhn. Ah. Ah,"

My mother interrupts, saying, "All right, Wilmer. Go to your cage."

I get into the cage very quickly, then stare at Christy, who is seated just outside the bars. She turns her head, looks at me, and sees me staring at her. She quickly looks away. I look away, too, but then look back. She partly turns her head back, looking now out of the corner of her eye, and again sees me staring at her. She averts her eyes. I do, too, but turn my gaze back again. After a moment, I reach out through the bars to touch her beautiful, store-bought coat.

She screams.

I scream.

My mother comes to calm me as Christy runs frantically out of the cabin. *Cut!*

We do this about ten times. I dread the Alka-Seltzer. It's up in my nose. It's burning my throat. I'm really thirsty. But soon it's all done. Hurray. Sigh of relief. Great job. We did it.

As we're leaving, everyone says, "I have a feeling we'll see you again!" *Christy* will air early next year and America will get its first look at Wilmer, peering out from under the table and scurrying to his cage.

Christy premiered on April 3, 1994. The show ran for two seasons. There were 20 episodes. Wilmer wasn't in any of them. Wilmer ended up on the cutting room floor.

I'll probably never know why they cut my part. Maybe it was just too much. Maybe having a screaming spastic dressed in rags, oatmeal, and peanut butter as a continuing character didn't fit in the same family-oriented genre as *Little House on the Prairie*. Maybe they felt that their target audience wouldn't respond favorably to such a frightening character. I don't know.

I imagine a series set in a holler in the Great Smoky Mountains of 1912 that tells about the life of a boy with dystonia. That would be gripping television, wouldn't it? I think I'll call it *Wilmer*.

Shortly after playing Wilmer, I read the book, *Frankenstein, The Modern Prometheus*, by Mary Shelley, first published in 1818. I was struck by how different it was from the iconic 1931 film that starred Boris Karloff. In the book, society's fear of Frankenstein makes him angry. In the movie, his brain, transplanted from a dead criminal, seals his fate from the start. Put another way, the book blames nurture, the movie blames nature. I prefer the original.

Frankenstein is a fixture in the consciousness of the modern world. Even small children know of his menacing presence. Frankenstein is the original and ultimate "other." My favorite portrayal is in *Young Frankenstein*, where Peter Boyle and Gene Wilder, the monster and his creator, put on the ritz and tap dance together in tuxedos. (Super-duper.) I think Mel Brooks had the right idea. Frankenstein was a charmer.

Storm Reading is going back on the road and I, of course, must go with it. I'm not as keen on touring as I once was. I know that sounds ungrateful, but it's hard for me to do. And besides, it's lonely, going from place to place, surrounded by strangers.

I have always wondered what it would be like to be married. Whenever I try to picture it, I see myself as more of a burden than a breadwinner. I'm almost 40, and even now I have no real job. A future? Not really. It seems that I'll always live in a world outside of the one I see others living in. Love? Somehow, it's not real. To me, insecurity is real.

I wonder again if someone with all these doubts and fears could ever be in a strong, committed relationship, never mind a marriage.

Still.

48
ALASKA CALLS

Jane Invites Me into Her Life

June 1994

The LAPD slowly follows O.J. Simpson up the 405.

Sheryl Crow is on the radio singing "All I Wanna Do."

~

RECENTLY, *STORM READING* has been performed on Sunset Boulevard, in an off-Broadway theater, and in Manchester, in the U.K.

We've been on the road for six months straight. It is less and less tolerable. The thrill has faded. It's more like a job now. A good job, to be sure, but still a job.

Right now, I'm in Anchorage, Alaska. I'm sitting near the front of the stage to interact with the audience after a near-perfect performance. From the audience, a woman directs a question to me. "Are you married?"

Gee. "N-n-n-no. I'm. Not." Oh, great. I sound like Billy in *Cuckoo's Nest*. But I'm absolutely thrilled. I have watched this scene play out a hundred times before, in films and on TV, but only now is its significance clear to me.

Here I am, 40 years old, and this is the first time in my life that I've been asked my marital status by someone who isn't a minor bureaucrat.

Afterwards, a woman with dark, graying hair comes backstage. "My name's Jane."

She's using a walker. Her hair flows over her shoulders. It's beautiful. "It's great to meet you." She's full of joy.

"Hi." I nod. No abrupt movements, now. She's quite attractive.

"I really loved your play. What are you doing tomorrow? Are you free?" She is looking for something, but who isn't? Steady now.

"Sure." That's better. One syllable, first try. She seems to be about my age. Maybe a little younger.

"I'd like to take you to see a glacier," she says. "I've got a car. Can I pick you up at your hotel?" Her look is direct, no shyness in it. She really is attractive.

"Okay," I say. "What time?" Be still, my flexing leg. I think I'd like to see this glacier.

~

She picks me up at six in the morning. The sun's already all the way up, but it's cloudy, and cold. In June. Welcome to Alaska.

We drive along an inlet for about an hour. On a grassy slope above us is a herd of Dall sheep. There is no fence between the car and these wild sheep. We turn down a road that ends near a lake. Since we left Anchorage, I think we've seen fewer than ten cars. We are alone out here, on a vast natural stage.

We get out and follow a paved trail to the lake's shore. Light, spring leaves fill the trees by the trail. There's no one else here. A few miles away, at the other end of the lake, is Portage Glacier, an ancient river of ice.

Jane tires quickly. She explains that it's because she has multiple sclerosis. I gallantly offer to push her in my chair, which she finds amusing. I offer to feed her, too, but she doesn't like that. A person only wants to accept so much help. Dependent, independent, and co-dependent. It is a delicate balance. We talk and walk. I think of asking her if multiple sclerosis is fatal, but I don't. Not now.

She asks me if I'd like to see her house. Of course! When we get there, she shows me her audition video for Very Special Arts. In it, she dances with her walker to the theme from "Flashdance … What a feeling!" If she is accepted, she will soon go to Europe with the VSA tour, performing and conducting seminars on disability and dance.

We talk for hours. I ask her about her MS, if it will worsen. She tells me that people do not usually die from MS. The talk turns into intimacy. She invites me. A rope has been lowered into the dark pit of my isolation.

Then we decide I shouldn't spend the night. I have to fly out tomorrow. She'll have to go to work. As we part at the hotel, we both promise to keep in touch.

Thinking back, I don't remember what we talked about. We just seemed to make each other smile and laugh from the start. She wasn't put off at all by my speech. It was as though we had been apart for a while and were catching up. From the start, we were testing our feelings about loving each other, and toward death. We were harmonizing.

It's late August now, I'm home. Jane went to Belgium with Very Special Arts. At a conference on disabilities in Berkeley, I performed a few scenes from my play and did a little improv. Ed Roberts was there. I roped his attendant into my act. She became the drive-through worker in the cheese-burger sketch. Ed smiled.

My sister, Wendy, helped me make the arrangements to meet Jane at a stopover in Seattle on her way home to Anchorage. The hotel was very helpful. Jane and I spent four wonderful days together in the room. Somewhere in there I asked her if she was the woman in the audience who asked me if I was married. She laughed and said she was.

Eric and Nora joined us for dinner on the last night of the stopover. The four of us made plans for adventures in Alaska.

49
MOSS ON PERMAFROST

Beyond the End of the Road and onto the Big Screen

August 1995
Christopher Reeve, who played Superman, is thrown from his horse.
Alison Hargreaves, the first woman to climb Mt. Everest without oxygen
or help from Sherpas, dies in an avalanche.

≈

ED ROBERTS PASSED away this spring. His memorial service was held in the Harmon Gym on the Berkeley campus. The gym couldn't hold all the people who showed up.

In March, Remy, Paul, and I performed my short piece, *The Art of Human Being*, at the Bay Area Dance Festival. At one point, Remy sat in my wheelchair and I sat on his lap. I was giving him lessons on how to be spastic. This is art. Thank you, Remy.

I'm in Anchorage.

I've been here with Jane since June. My place in Berkeley is vacant. Wendy moved out for now. This morning, Eric and Nora left for Seattle. For the past week, the four of us have been traveling together in Alaska, a place with almost no fences. It is rugged. It is wild. Out here, we are beyond the fence. Out here, we are free.

Our best adventure was the trip to Grasshopper Valley.

To get there, first we have to drive to the end of a road about fifty miles from Anchorage. Then we fly up a wide river valley in a small, loud plane designed for very short, rough airstrips. There's not enough room for all four of us, so Eric and I go first. On the flight out, we see no sign of human life. Nothing but green valleys, white glaciers, and snow-capped mountains. The pilot points out a mother bear and her cubs running along a slope below. The river becomes a glacier that we follow for miles, then we turn sharply north, drop suddenly, steeply, into a narrow, glacier-carved valley with mile-high walls. The valley is several miles long, running north to south. Each end of the valley is blocked by a wall of ice. Our stomachs are in our mouths, and *thump!* We bump along briefly, then come to an abrupt stop.

I get out of the plane, and I am in another world. I just flew over miles of ice and, here, the sun is shining and a light breeze is blowing off the glacier to the south. There are scores of waterfalls running down steep rocky slopes and onto the green curve of the foothills that end in the river in front of me. The valley floor is decorated with patches of brush and stands of saplings, all surrounded by a carpet of thick, rich moss interrupted by patches of pebbly sand. I take off my shoes and sink my feet into the moss. I take off my shirt.

Dave helps unload our gear and shows us around the camp. There are three tents: two for sleeping, one for cooking. The reason for this division of purpose becomes clear when Dave discovers that the big tin of ground coffee has been raided by bears. It is all gone. I did not know that bears like coffee. Dave seems neither surprised nor worried. Without meaning to, I imagine a family of bears hopped up on caffeine. He tells us not to panic if we encounter a bear and, whatever else we do, not to run. I assure him I won't.

He shows us the camp's two three-wheeled, metal-framed wheelchairs with pull bars. They were designed by a guy who wanted to ascend Kilimanjaro but couldn't walk. Then Dave warns us that the weather can change suddenly around glaciers and that if he can't land when he comes back with Nora and Jane, that we shouldn't worry, he'll drop us food and other supplies. This, I believe, is meant to reassure us. With that, he gets back in the plane, taxis less than a quarter mile north to the end of the rocky airstrip, turns around, revs the engine with the brakes on, then takes off with a roar. Dave is already airborne as he passes us. Eric and I are left alone with our thoughts.

Eric turns to me and says, "I don't have to be able to outrun a bear, I only have to be able to outrun you." We both laugh.

Dave returns with Jane and Nora about an hour later. No food drop today. He helps them get out, unloads some more gear, says he'll be back in two days, then, *roar!* We're alone. In Eden.

Jane and I look at the moss. I look at Jane. Jane looks at me. She says, "It's beautiful here!"

"Yeah!" I think we are both having the same thought.

Eric and Nora wheel us to the middle of a giant green pillow of moss under a distant canopy of the purest, deepest blue. They head back to the tents with strict instructions to return in three hours. And not a minute less.

A blanket spread out on undulating velvety moss by the glacier. Not far below us, permafrost, perpetually frozen ground. Around us, the rustle and shimmer of cottonwood saplings in the breeze that both warms and cools. Bobwhites call. I am in Shangri-la.

At the end of the summer, Jane comes to visit me here in Berkeley.

She brought me a goofy moose hand puppet with antlers made of twigs. The weather is nice this December, but not too warm. This is important, because warm weather makes her MS worse. Jane calls it "melting." I have borrowed a power chair for her from a friend, so we can roam the city in comfort and style.

Telegraph Avenue is lined with booths for the annual Street Fair. Herbal teas. Handmade soap. Tie-dyed scarves. Indian jewelry. Carved driftwood. Just the basics. My friend Brenda, who is making a coffee table book about disabled people and sex, invites us to a photoshoot, where we strike a few romantic poses. Brenda is on the cutting edge of creating disability culture. We met when she came to see my play, *My Sexual History*.

Most nights Jane and I dine out with friends, usually at Italian restaurants in Berkeley. I now consider dining out to be a political act. It is revolutionary, an unashamed public declaration of a simple human right. It is also great fun. One evening, we go to a dance jam and dance together on the floor.

$\sim$

It's mid-January now and I'm staying at a little inn near the Lobero Theatre in Santa Barbara.

I went to Anchorage over Christmas and caught a cold. I still ache all over. I'm exhausted. Like I'm underwater. And there's this lump on my neck. It's sore. I'm putting ice on it. I really should be at home in Berkeley, resting in bed, but I can't take any time off from the show. Not now.

I'm about to become a movie star. After a seven-year run, the last two performances of *Storm Reading* will be filmed in front of a live audience here at the Lobero. Four cameras will record everything. We're in rehearsal now. Curtain's up in four days.

I have a confession to make. For a long time I felt like I was pretending. Pretending to be an artist. Pretending to be a poet, a writer, a dancer, a playwright, an actor. Kurt Vonnegut said, "We are what we pretend to be, so we must be careful what we pretend to be." Well, Mr. Vonnegut, the rehearsals were hard. I'm not feeling much better. But the show must go on. And I know I'm not pretending now.

The curtain goes up for the first performance. I go out. The audience is full of energy. Things are going pretty well, but toward the end, it's like I'm running out of gas. I fumble a line. My legs shake. My neck hurts. Another line. I gasp for breath. I actually fall once. But it doesn't seem to matter. At the end, everyone is pleased. A standing ovation. Curtain calls.

The following day we shoot closeups of individual scenes, without an audience. To get the shots that are hard to get when it's live. The director says that last night's performance was really just a dress rehearsal. Tonight we have to be in sync. Everything has to be right. Tonight will be the final performance of *Storm Reading*.

In the darkness of the wings, just before I go on, I once again extend the index finger of my right hand and touch the flattened penny, still taped to the armrest of my chair. The one my father placed on the railroad track so long ago. My good luck piece.

I'm on.

~

We nailed it. One of our best. In the morning we pile in the van. On the way home, we pull over to watch as surfers share a wave with a school of dolphins hurtling toward the shore, backlit by the morning sun.

50
Mountain Climbing

We Travel into the Wilderness Together

Summer 1997

The most-watched American television series is *ER*.

"Goodbye England's Rose" becomes the best-selling single in history.

∼

In January, Remy Charlip and I celebrated our birthdays together at a big bash in the lobby of my building. I turned 43, Remy, 68. Lots of food. Lots of stories. My mom did some improv.

A young woman performed Remy's piece, *Dance in a Winged Chair*. This dance is special to me. It says that you can dance without moving, that a chair is a stage, that nothing is every bit as real as something, and that you can interpret anything in infinite ways.

In March, the movie *Breathing Lessons: The Life and Work of Mark O'Brien,* won an Academy Award for Best Documentary. Jessica Yu won the Oscar, but Mark was the star.

∼

I am in Anchorage.

Well, we're just going to have to do it on our own. Everybody we asked to go with us is busy. Jane and I are going to drive into the heart of the Alaskan wilderness and camp.

There are a few practical considerations. Jane can't walk and is, quite literally, losing her grip. She can still manipulate the hand controls on the van, though, so she's the designated driver. While I can't really walk either, I can get from here to there. Combine this with the fact that my grip is, if anything, too firm, and I am the designated arms and legs of this operation. Jane got a neighbor to fold down the back seat of the van and install a foam mattress. She also got help filling a six-gallon water jug under the back seat. We can do this, if I can just figure out how to get these sleeping bags zipped.

On Thursday afternoon we head out. North of Palmer, we head west through Hatcher Pass, and on into the mountains beyond. We take the right fork of the road into a gigantic trough scooped out by a glacier during the last ice age. Archangel Valley.

The map shows that we are only three miles from the campsite at the end of the road. Should be easy, right? No. The Japanese engineers who designed this van were thinking of the smooth pavement of the highway from Tokyo to Kyoto, not the dirt and gravel of the Archangel Valley Road, with gaping potholes every two or three feet, many of them deeper than the tires of our van. This could become a serious problem. Picture a tire hanging suspended in a pothole. I believe the technical term is "high-centered." Jane's number one job is now to avoid these deep potholes. To do this, she must successfully maneuver the van into and out of the lesser potholes, ever-so-carefully finding a safe path into the mountains. And this she does, masterfully. Yes, the van scrapes and grinds against the rocks of the road, but an hour or so later, we arrive at the end of the road.

We are surrounded by broken mountain tops. It is stunning. Now if we can just turn this thing around. Jane cuts the wheels and slowly backs up to get us pointed the way we came. The soil on the edge of the road is soft, though, and the rear of the van begins to sink, slipping slowly toward a massive ditch. Jane pushes the accelerator with her hand, but the wheels spin as the rear of the van inches further into the ditch.

Oh. My. God.

In my mind's eye, I see rescue helicopters hovering, lowering metal baskets to helmeted men in orange jumpsuits with arms outstretched.

Then Jane throws it into reverse.

Now.

I am not what you would call an experienced driver. I do know quite a lot about golf carts and electric wheelchairs, sure, but driving Japanese vans in the Alaskan wilderness is outside my area of expertise. That does not prevent me from having opinions about wilderness van driving, however, and, to me, with my limited experience, to put a van in reverse when it is sliding backward into a muddy king-sized ditch seems counterintuitive.

In reverse now, the van backs a foot or so farther into the ditch. Then Jane deftly puts it in low with one hand while gunning it with the other and, *voila*! The van pops up onto the road. Just like that. Good thing I wasn't driving. We'd be riding home in a chopper.

Ever so carefully, Jane parks the van on the edge of the road, a respectful distance from the waiting ditch.

This entire journey is a series of little victories. Society tells us that we are "severely disabled." Society expects us to stay at home, or in "a home." Somewhere safe, where help is just a call or a buzz away. There was a time when people like us didn't go anywhere without a lot of help. But here we are. We are alone in these mountains. We got here by ourselves, without a lot of help. We have come where no couple like us has come before. We are breaking new ground here, in the middle of nowhere, at the end of the road in Archangel Valley. Sort of like Lewis and Clark. This is historic.

To be clear, then. I'm not free because I'm "disabled." I am free because I'm me. And while I cannot "climb mountains," I can climb mountains.

In the morning, I awaken on a moonlike terrain, my sweetheart by my side. I've always dreamed of this. We made it. We're like the first people on the moon. And our spaceship is intact. I get out of the van. There is even life here. In the stream, below the shoulder of the road, a beaver family has built a lodge. One is swimming silently below the surface. Other than that, we're alone, with no one else but God. We make love, then sleep, then make love again.

Watching the clouds move, the silence is incredible. It is deafening at first, then seems to listen. Jagged, rugged peaks and great chunks of craggy wet rock are all around, with patches and swathes of bright green moss everywhere, sending in roots that slowly grind away, patiently turning solid rock into potting soil. All it needs is time. There is a great power in these peaks. A strength that slows time to a crawl and dispels illusion.

51
A Network Opening

This is the Big Time

March 1998

Google will start up in the fall.

***Titanic* has been nominated for Best Picture.**

I'VE BEEN AT LOOSE ends, hanging out in Berkeley since *Storm Reading* closed. It was a huge part of my life.

Jane is home in Anchorage, still working, but slowly getting weaker. With MS, first the insulation around the nerve dissolves, then the nerve stops working. It often starts in the hands and feet, then works its way up. Jane has been getting more numb, and more paralyzed. I'm going to go see her in a few months. I miss her. But I don't really want to think about it. About what lies ahead. I'm feeling pretty lost.

I'm at home, preparing a talk about disability culture that I'm delivering tomorrow at the University. I suggest that we use art to grab people's attention, to engage them more deeply than is possible with intellect alone.

Truth wrapped in beauty can be irresistible. My notes are almost done. The phone rings.

"Hello."

"Hi, Neil. This is Tony. Tony Edwards." Which means Anthony Edwards, who produced and directed the documentary *Speaking Through Walls* and who is now one of the stars of *ER*, NBC's hit series. My mind stops its other operations and focuses on this one question: why is Anthony Edwards calling me? *Gulp.*

"Hi."

"Hey, Neil. We've got a great story on *ER* with a really sweet part in it for you. The character is a guy with cerebral palsy who needs medical attention but has trouble being understood. It's perfect for you. Are you available?"

"I'm. In!"

I have a thousand questions, but don't ask them, not wanting to give the impression that I am in any way hesitant. I will also wait to mention that I have dystonia, not cerebral palsy. Wouldn't want to miss this big break.

"Great! I'll mail you the script!"

After he hangs up, I reflect a bit. I understand that I am a disabled person and that the show is looking for a real disabled person to play the role of a disabled character. That's a good thing, a step in the right direction. Even ten years ago, they would have automatically hired a non-disabled actor for this role. Like Al Jolson, in blackface.

I think that a disabled person acting is not just an actor but also a symbol of the continuing struggle for liberation. A disabled person on the screen is a statement in itself. As more disabled people appear on the screen, as we gather a greater audience, things will change for the better. A new normal. I just hope my part portrays disability positively.

∼

I finally got the script in the mail. I had already gone to the lobby to check the mailbox three times.

My character is Mr. Lorenzo, the world's foremost authority on, get this, deciphering hieroglyphics. Ha! He's a successful academic with cerebral palsy who is admitted to the ER after being hit by a car. This is not your stereotypical movie version of the disabled victim. The script now reads that Mr. Lorenzo "babbles and jabbers" unintelligibly, but Tony has already assured me that Mr. Lorenzo, unlike Wilmer, will have actual spoken lines. The writers are already working on them.

It's March 12. Teresa from NBC calls to make all the arrangements. I get Eric on the phone. Shirt, pants, and shoe sizes. Check. Make sure my clothes are consistent with Chicago weather in spring. Got it. Join the Screen Actors Guild. Okay. Gee, I've got to figure out all the implications of getting a fat paycheck. Limo to and from both airports. First class air, round-trip. Limo to and from the hotel. Wow. Okay. Adjoining room with Eric and Nora, who will fly from Arizona to help out. Good. Rental car for the duration of the shoot. Perfect. Yes, the Hilton will be fine. Teresa will call back with all the details.

ER was created by Michael Crichton, who wrote *The Andromeda Strain* and *Jurassic Park*. In addition to Anthony Edwards, it stars George Clooney and Noah Wyle. All three of them have been nominated for Emmys. The show itself won the Peabody award. Last week, *ER* was number one in the Nielsen ratings, with more than 30 million viewers, far more than any other series. If *Storm Reading* was a cannon to get people's attention, *ER* is an intercontinental ballistic missile. Appearing on *ER* is not just an opportunity, it's a huge responsibility.

ER is shot in the emergency room of the County General Hospital in Chicago, Illinois. There's a covered entrance where ambulances pull up, automatic doors that open for the gurney. A waiting room with fiberglass chairs bolted to metal frames, vending machines and a bulletin board festooned with notices of various colors. A reception and triage area. Examination and consultation rooms. Trauma and operating rooms. Offices. An elevator.

But if you open the venetian blinds on the windows in the hospital administrator's office, you will not see the Chicago skyline or even a hospital corridor. No. The office window looks into an operating room. Nice view. And if you turn right at the reception counter instead of left, you're in what looks like a cavernous warehouse with a huge buffet table covered with mounds of snacks. It is like you've stepped into *The Twilight Zone*. Get in the elevator and push the button to take you to the second floor, and you've got a long wait ahead of you. This elevator doesn't move. The only thing that works on this elevator is the door. And the little lights and bells.

That's because you're in a one-story building. With no basement. It is a fake elevator. In a fake emergency room. There's no such thing as County General Hospital. You're not even in Chicago. You're in Burbank, California, at Warner Brothers Studios. On Stage 3.

Each episode of *ER* costs 13 million dollars. They make 22 every year. One in every ten people in the United States will watch my story when it is broadcast in April. Then it will be aired internationally. Then there will be reruns. People all over the world will hear Mr. Lorenzo's story.

ER is a very big deal.

〜

Mr. Lorenzo is brought to the ER after being hit by a car. He has abrasions and lacerations. His clothes are cut away to allow rapid examination and diagnosis. It's nothing serious, nothing that even requires that he be admitted to the hospital. But the admitting physician, played by Noah Wyle, assumes that Mr. Lorenzo's problems with speech and movement were caused by the accident. "Can you open your hand?" he asks, gently tugging on the fingers of Mr. Lorenzo's right fist. Needless to say, the fingers remain curled. The hospital gears up to do a whole battery of tests to determine whether emergency brain surgery is indicated. Mr. Lorenzo's repeated efforts to explain himself are either ignored or misunderstood. Eventually, however, a nurse figures out that the patient is actually talking and making sense. In the end, the admitting physician apologizes for not taking the time to listen to what Mr. Lorenzo was trying to say.

All of this is accomplished with only a minimal reliance on sanctioned pity, soothed guilt, shameless self-promotion, or morbid curiosity.

On the one hand, Mr. Lorenzo's tale is just another sub-plot from another soap opera. Like *General Hospital,* but more posh. On the other hand, it is much more than that. This is a modern myth being told around the electronic campfire to the global tribe. This is how the consciousness of humanity is shaped. When the myth changes, the consciousness changes. And the moral of this story is simple: don't jump to conclusions about people based on irrelevant differences. More broadly: don't judge people. More narrowly: people with disabilities are entitled to respect, dignity, and positive expectations. Everyone is. My hope is that Mr. Lorenzo's story will create more positive expectations all around.

On the set, I was treated as a fellow professional actor. I was treated with respect and dignity, and all the expectations people had of me were quite positive. I returned the favor.

Thank you, Tony. And thank you, Noah.

Right after I got back to Berkeley, Jane's friend Fran called me. Jane was in the hospital, she said. She also said that she thought Jane's time was just about up.

I put myself on the next flight to Anchorage.

5²
DRIFT

(Jane)

April 1998

~

JANE.

You are asleep in a hospital bed in Providence Hospital in Anchorage.

I am sitting by your side in a "loaner" wheelchair. It's cold outside. The trees are still bare. Spring comes late here. I've been staying at the Ronald McDonald House near the hospital.

You have pneumonia.

When you were admitted, you were barely breathing and had hypothermia. I'm pretty sure it was because you kept your house so cold. I know it helps your MS, but this time you were too cold for too long. Fran had gone by your house and found you. As soon as they brought you in, they piled blankets on you and did everything they could to get your body temperature up, but it stayed at 86 for a long time. Fran said you were mumbling and rambling. One thing you said to the staff was that your boyfriend was on the TV show *ER*. Fran said they thought you were out of your head.

They put you in intensive care and hooked you up to all kinds of tubes and hoses. When I showed up, no one asked if I was the mysterious boyfriend. They assumed I was another patient. They were jumping to conclusions. Mr. Lorenzo's episode of *ER* won't be on until the end of the month.

When they moved you to progressive care, I came to your room. You were having a lot of trouble breathing. A whistling sound.

"How long?" you asked. You were still very confused. "Am I awake?" I was worried. "I don't want to wake up." I didn't want to be a burden to you, so I sat outside your door, watching people walk back and forth. No one questioned my right to be there. It was as though I had a hall pass.

Three days later I heard you ask, "Where's Neil?" I came in. You looked exhausted, but not confused. You smiled at me and said, "Look what a mess I've gotten myself into. I've been trying to control everything about my life for a long time, trying to manipulate things so that my MS wasn't so obvious. I was trying to hide it. What a mess." Then you told me about the circle of life and how all of this is happening for a reason and that the reason is love. I did not disagree.

I started visiting you every day. I got over my fear. I was good at not needing to talk. I just sat with you. Several days later, you told me you loved me. You asked me to promise I'd keep living my life. I said I loved you. I promised.

Then you fell asleep. You slept for hours. When you woke up, you were stronger. You asked for your gown. You accepted medication. It was like your system had rebooted.

You were permitted to take liquids. Quick, brusque sponge baths were administered by nursing assistants discussing late house payments. People talked to you in the high, loud voice usually reserved for puppies, children, and people with dementia. And still you grew stronger.

When they told you that you would be moved to a skilled nursing facility, you took it very well. What had once been your worst nightmare suddenly seemed like a step toward freedom.

In mid-May, you were admitted to Our Lady of Compassion, a nursing home. It was better than the hospital, but it wasn't home. Several of your friends were wrestling with stubborn bureaucracies to make it possible for you to once again live in your own home. Home is where you wanted to be.

❧

It is June now. Your friends prevail. You go home. Home to quiet, privacy, and home cooking, with an assistant around the clock. It's still not easy, but you are free.

I, on the other hand, am having a hard time. My body is tighter than usual, more clenched. Maybe the stress of the hospital and nursing home is getting to me. I am drained of energy. I have aches and pains that won't go away. In my neck. In my joints. I can't sleep. With you settled in at home now, I go back to Berkeley for rest and recuperation. Wendy moves in again to help me. She's more eager to help me than I am to receive it, but I am grateful, and I accept it. I don't like needing help. But I do.

❧

It's September now. I feel a bit better and I'm back with Jane at her house in Anchorage. She is much weaker. I do my best to be there for her. She still has a full-time attendant. We are hoping for the best.

When James Cameron's *Titanic* hit the theaters, I didn't go. I somehow knew that it might hit too close to home. When it came out in video, someone gave it to Jane. What could I do? We started watching it together.

A little way into it, Jane turned to me and told me she was having trouble with her eyes. She asked me if it would be okay if I finished the movie alone.

Her vision has been failing for some time. MS can do that. But she also may have figured out where this story was headed.

It took quite a while to get Jane put to bed, even with an attendant. When everything was set, I went back out to the living room to watch the rest of the movie. I was hooked, but I couldn't stand to watch too much at a time. After a scene or two, I went to see how Jane was doing. She asked me how the movie was going. I sighed heavily and said, "This. Is. Very. Hard. To. Take."

The same thing happened several times more, over several nights. And it got harder and harder to take. Winslet and DiCaprio, clinging to the debris in the darkness, far from shore. A monumental love that was fated to come to a tragic end.

Fiction colliding with non-fiction on the cold night sea.

It's now the end of September. Jane is not herself. The connections with reality that we take for granted are coming undone. She is asking herself basic questions: where am I? How did I get here? When is this? And she is no longer knows the answers. So she asks me. I answer and she nods, reassured. Then, a while later, she asks me the same questions again. Who are you? Soon, my answers fail to orient her at all. Then she stops asking. She has forgotten the questions altogether. She has come unmoored.

I'm weak. It's early November. Winter's coming. It's cold. My bones ache. My neck hurts all the time. I can't sleep. Jane has assistants to take care of her. I'd better take care of myself. My love is not strong enough.

I have to go home.

Jane.

You are a climber on Everest, gasping for life near the top of the world. Disabled people live very close to the sky. They keep warm with cloaks and scarves and thermoses filled with hot broth. Each step is put into the footprint of those who went before, measuring time and distance. At five miles high, the air is thin. The mind begins to wander. The winds rise up to gale force. The terrain becomes solid white. No up or down. In the middle of nowhere. Look up there. I think the summit is just beyond that crest. Tomorrow, we won't have far to go. If the weather is clear, it'll be easy.

We'll be able to take our time.

~

On December 5, 1998, Jane passed away in Providence Hospital.

The sand had run out.

53
LIVING SPIRITS

Mastering the Art of *Butoh*

1999

Vladimir Putin is gathering the reins of power in Russia.
Neo learns about the matrix from Morpheus.

DURING THE TWENTY years I've lived in Berkeley, my circle of friends has grown steadily. My appearance on *ER,* however, seems to have made me into something of a local celebrity. Before, I knew lots of people that I met socially or through cultural events in the area. Now, many more people know me on sight, and some of them feel they have a special bond with me.

While I still feel a bit wary of people, it is good to be seen, to be known. It makes society feel more like a family, much warmer than the cold world described by Blind Chuck. When I roll up Telegraph Avenue, people's faces often light up with smiles. No one is invisible.

Wendy moved out of the spare room a while ago and returned to her home up north. It's nice to know that whenever I need help, Wendy is there. Sometimes she drives me a little nuts, but life is harder without her here to help.

I flew to Anchorage to attend a dance at the University of Alaska, the last work choreographed by Jane. All of her friends were there.

Mark O'Brien died. Complications from bronchitis.

Back in Berkeley, I watched a live, televised performance of Mikhail Baryshnikov's White Oak Project. At 51 years old, he is considered ancient for ballet. I'm 45 and sympathize.

Now that *Storm Reading* is over, I am dancing more.

Recently, I learned about *butoh*, a form of dance theater created in Japan by Tatsumi Hijikata. A friend had given me a wrinkled photocopy of a book translated from Japanese. I was lying on my bed, flipping through the coffee-stained pages, when a passage caught my eye. I recall he said something like this: "When I began to wish I were crippled, even though I am perfectly healthy, or rather when I thought I would have been better off had I been born a cripple, that is the first step towards *butoh*."

Had Mr. Hijikata created a form of dance rooted in disability? This I had to see.

I learned that the *butoh* company Harupin-Ha is right here in Berkeley. It was founded twenty years ago by Hijikata's first students, Koichi and Hiroko Tamano. They brought *butoh* to the Americas. Last night, for the first time, I saw the Tamanos perform.

A single performer covered in white, both costume and makeup, steps onto a bare stage as an untuned, arhythmic *samisen* plays. The performer's movements are uncoordinated, disjointed, sometimes spastic. Then he flails. He looks malformed and crippled. His face is a sequence of exaggerated expressions, some that correspond to no known human emotion. He is strange, possessed, even unearthly. He is an angular marionette with no one holding the strings. A zombie. A robot. An alien hand puppet of the life force. Otherworldly.

I said, "Wow. This. Includes. Me. My. Body. Type. My. Aesthetic." I had long suspected that there could be an identifiable disability aesthetic, just as there are other aesthetics, like punk and goth. Looked at this way, the aesthetic is not so much about disability as it is about art itself. Like cubism, or surrealism. Like a Jackson Pollock painting.

I learned more about the origins of *butoh*, how, after World War II, Japan struggled to awaken from a nightmare. Cities in ashes, people destitute, myths shattered. A few performance artists felt that existing traditional dance forms could not express the post-traumatic inner life of this new, post-Hiroshima Japan, so they created a new form that could.

At first, *butoh* celebrated the squat and earthy movements of the Japanese farmer working the land, thumbing its nose at the refined and genteel notions of an elite aesthetic tradition rooted in the feudal past. Geishas in kimonos were replaced by peasants in rags. It drew from the uncouth, the coarse, and the taboo side of daily rural life and felt a kinship with the rebellious avant-garde movement that emerged from the rubble in post-war Europe. Then it grew wider, to include any authentic expression of the life force that was stripped of the artificial constructs and conventions of traditional dance, drama, and music.

The creative latitude of *butoh* means that it is, in principle, open to everyone. You don't need a symmetrical body with long, sculpted muscles. In fact, not having that perfect symmetry, not having that smooth coordination that is so essential to graceful classical movement, can be an asset. And you don't have to spend years stretching, jumping and spinning, or practicing predetermined moves and ritualized routines. While these may be prerequisites to achieving the ethereal grace in a *pas de deux*, they are not needed to channel the life force.

This is not to say that *butoh* is easy. Pushing your body to its brink is common in *butoh* exercise. Try it. Strike the pose of a driftwood stump with its sun-bleached toes rooted in the sand at the high tide line. Now hold it, while pushing a baby buggy through a field of stars.

You don't need a perfectly aligned wrist to grasp the divine fire.

The dance scene in and around San Francisco is open to everyone. It includes every kind of dance from all over the world and welcomes innovation. Tradition coexists and mixes with the novel, the experimental. Purists compete with iconoclasts in a lively scene that constantly changes. I become part of that change.

I plunge into this world, seeking out performance opportunities at festivals, workshops, and other events. One consequence of my performing is that the people in the audience become accustomed to seeing dancers with disabilities on stage. People who once raised their eyebrows in surprise or even amusement at the suggestion that they should watch a spastic dance come to these events, see me dance, and realize that able dancers do not enjoy a monopoly on beauty and truth.

I was so very lucky to have found *butoh*. Its emphasis on imperfection rather than perfection, the opposite of classical ballet, suits me. Its movements, like mine, have nothing to do with *Swan Lake*. And I'm not sure that *butoh* is merely a form of dance. It may be more than an aesthetic, too. It seems to contain a philosophy, and a sort of politics as well. Whatever it is, it fits very well with my spastic dancing, and with the social reality of being disabled. And what a rare and wonderful thing that is.

Christina Braun, an accomplished practitioner of *butoh*, and I performed together in a garden surrounded by a score of sculptures by Auguste Rodin, who created "The Thinker" and "The Kiss." Gary Ivanek filmed it. With encouragement, a few members of the audience became part of the performance. It was pretty wild.

With an extended arm of many angles. I dance to uncover truth. Life is a dance. This life. With a turn of the head, posed with purpose, eyes squeezed closed. This is art. And when I dance, I am visible, on stage, bare-chested, my wings bend upward in stars. From foot to sky.

I dance to say things that are beyond words. It is a way of saying, "Look. Look here. I am an important part of the universe. Look at this part of the universe. It is like no other."

I am art.

⁓

I need a break, a vacation. I go with Eric and Norah to Cayman. The highlight of the trip is snorkeling in the middle of a school of friendly giant, puppy-like, stingrays. I swim among them with an innertube around my chest and my masked face in the water. I hold them in my arms. It is like being in another world.

The warm water eases my pain.

54
ANOTHER ROUNDABOUT

I Ease My Aching Neck

2001

An international team decodes the human genome.
Later this year, two Boeing 767s will be deliberately flown into
the World Trade Center.

~

I'M ON MY BED IN Berkeley. With a sore neck. As a rule, I don't talk to people about my medical problems. It's boring, gruesome, and no good comes from it. But now I'm going to break that rule, not because I want sympathy but because I want you to understand this part of what it means to be disabled, to have dystonia. The medical part. I want you to be able to glimpse it from my point of view.

~

I'm 47. I can't hop anymore. Walking has become almost impossible. All of my muscles feel weak, drained of energy, as though they're completely exhausted. And my limbs feel tingly, like electricity is trickling through them. My sister Wendy moves back into the spare room to help out. She takes me to the doctor.

My neurologist takes one look at the MRI of my neck and says, "Oh, damn."

In the world of medicine, these words rarely bode well. Then she says, "This is not good."

See? I told you.

"There's been quite a change since the last time."

I brace myself.

"I'm sorry, buddy, but your spinal cord is being crushed."

I find myself wondering if she has ever called a patient with a spinal cord that was not being crushed "buddy," then ask myself whether focusing on this infantilizing endearment should be my highest priority just now.

"I'm setting you up with a neurosurgeon right now. Time is of the essence."

More than 35 years ago, Dr. Rosner told my parents and me that dystonia can be really hard on a body. He told us that it is hardest on the joints. Where the bones meet. He was right.

The disc that serves as a cushion between two of my neck bones has been squeezed out of place by the constant involuntary flexing of my powerful neck muscles. Making matters worse, there is a hole in that disc. It leaks. This dislocation and rupture is putting pressure on my spinal cord. In addition, the two neck bones are now rubbing together, bone on bone. Grating. The ensuing inflammation has added to the pressure on my spinal cord. There's even a bony lump on one of the neck bones that is scraping the sheath of the spinal cord. Not good. They call the pressure on the spinal cord 'stenosis'. It hurts.

Worse than that, though, is that when there is too much pressure on the spinal cord, it can't do its job as well. It can't carry signals from the brain to the body effectively. This is causing my arms and legs to feel weak, making it hard for me to move them with any force.

The really bad news is that, if this continues, I may end up not being able to move my arms and legs at all. I may be paralyzed. Quadriplegic. It could even become irreversible. Permanent.

It has been suggested by a team of doctors that I have a procedure. They want to cut open my throat, take out the ruptured disc, remove the bony lump, then fuse the two neck bones together with screws. And then, of course, sew me back up.

So. Not much of a choice.

On July 15, 2001, at the hospital before surgery, I take out the photograph of the Warner Bros lot with me and George Clooney who plays a doctor on *ER*. I show it to the group of doctors, nurses, and medical technicians who attend to me. They all smile and relax and say, "Really? That's so cool," and things like that. My intention is to encourage them to see me as a real person, not as a medical subject, a specimen. And, to be frank, I want them to see me as a person with status, not as the equivalent of an untouchable in the American caste system. As Jesse Jackson would say, "I am somebody." I become visible to them. I become a person. I pass out copies of the picture. They perform the procedure. They fuse my neck bones together.

The surgery is over. I'm on my bed and my neck really hurts. A friend calls to tell me about an article he read. He says they've found a cure for dystonia.

55

THE TOUCH OF TECHNOLOGY

Shocking Rogue Brain Cells

May 2003

The space shuttle *Columbia* disintegrates upon re-entry.

The One Ring That Rules Them All is destroyed in the Cracks

of Doom in Mordor.

MY NECK FEELS BETTER now. It's still a bit stiff and sore, but the stenosis seems to be gone. My arms and legs are strong again, and back to performing energetic, if unauthorized, maneuvers.

Brain surgeons don't freeze brain cells anymore. Science has marched on. These days, when they want to tweak dystonia, they zap the rogue brain cells with a little jolt of electricity. It is called deep brain stimulation, or DBS. To get at the insubordinate brain cells, two electrode wires are threaded into the brain and left there. A battery about the size of a really thick half-dollar provides the power. The battery is tucked under the skin below the collarbone with wires leading to the electrodes. The zap is when the electrons jump from the end of one electrode to the other. They aren't really sure how it all works, but it often does, and the zapped brain cells don't die, as they do when frozen.

So. It has been suggested that I let a team of doctors put electrodes deep inside my brain. This is not the kind of permission that one grants without some serious thought. The team sent me a great deal of information to ponder, including videos of people with dystonia who had the procedure and are now spasm-free. I watched these videos. The before and after clips. No more spasms. I reviewed the data. As with all surgical procedures, there are risks, and there are no guarantees. But what catches my eye are the videos. Before and after. No spasms.

Now.

In my little corner of the world, this is headline news. Practically speaking, DBS can be said to sometimes cure dystonia. Without killing any brain cells.

You might think that I would be eager to give the go-ahead, but it's not that simple. For almost forty years, I have been locked up in spasm prison. I have been shaped by dystonia, both physically and psychologically. My body and my mind. I have adjusted to its demands. I execute strategies for living that take into account dystonia's costs and benefits. My expectations are calibrated on a dystonic scale. Even my rationalizations are built on the bedrock of dystonia. Look, dystonia has not prevented me from finding personal and professional success. And I have met countless people who do not have dystonia who aren't as happy as I am. I have lived successfully with dystonia for 40 years. I'm good at it.

But when someone holds out the prospect of a cure, right there, under my nose, all the carefully crafted strategies, the finely calibrated expectations, and the field-tested cost-benefit analyses fly out the window. The stark light of hope can defrock a rationalization more quickly and thoroughly than any amount of logic or evidence.

Suddenly, there it is, front and center, the question that I dared to ask aloud only when I was a child, and then only once. The question that I cannot afford to ask.

"When will I be better?"

Can't they see how unbelievably cruel it is to dangle hope in front of me like this? *Not* hoping has been a cornerstone of my successful life. *Not* hoping has kept me sane these 40 years. I clearly remember how I felt when I went into remission. Now, like then, I don't dare hope. I can't hope that DBS will stop the spasms, the way it did for the people in the videos. I just can't. But, here's the thing, I can't *not* hope, either. I can't. Hope sucks, all around.

"We can help," say the neurosurgeons.

I have met a lot of neurosurgeons. They are fine people. But there's something about the profession that attracts a certain kind of person. They're quite competitive. It seems like you can't really be a brain surgeon unless you like sports. During various procedures, I've heard them talking about the sports they like to play, about their games of golf, tennis, and paddleball. It's clear they relish a good match. And over time, I've learned that one of their favorite sports is surgery itself. They keep score. How good they are at surgery determines their wealth, and, more importantly, their prestige. They each want to be the Michael Jordan of the operating table. I can see it in their eyes. They want to win.

And what is my role in this sport? Am I a player? No. I'm assigned the position of the ever-patient patient, supine on the operating table. Powerless. Helpless. Actually, it's worse than that. In this blood sport, I'm the playing field.

What is help? They don't know. I'm sure of it. But, fair enough. I know. And I get to decide what happens here. It is up to me. Because I am the Kareem Abdul-Jabbar of a country called Disabled. And I alone will decide whether they get to play their game at all.

One more thing. The struggle to end the oppression of disabled people is like a battle and the disabled people fighting for the cause are its soldiers. I know this because I have been in the trenches of this battle for decades. Viewed this way, a cure is not as completely innocent as it sounds. It contains an element of betrayal.

On May 19, 2003, I once again handed out pictures of George Clooney and me. Smiles all around. A young nurse in blue scrubs says, "That's so awesome! I just love him!" Then a team of surgeons placed electrodes deep in my brain.

And.

It didn't work. The spasms continued, unabated. And then I got an infection from the surgery. But wait, there's more. One of the electrodes inside my brain broke.

Let's just say that the procedure was not a rip-roaring success.

After the surgery, the University of California contacted me and asked if they could archive my papers in the Bancroft Library. I filled six banker's boxes with drawings, newsletters, newspaper clippings, correspondence, and medical records. I also taught a class at Berkeley with Susan Schweik called "Disability and Digital Storytelling."

I'm 49 now. The pain inside my right hip has been getting worse. Okay, it's severe.

56
THE KICK BOXING EFFECT
I Try to Ease My Aching Hip

October 2003

James Gandolfini wins an Emmy for his role as Tony Soprano.
Data from the WMAP satellite suggest that the universe
is 13.7 billion years old.

THROUGH THE DECADES, my right hip joint has been subjected to as much stress as that of a fat Ukrainian folk dancer. My right leg has the habit of lying low until the least appropriate moment then suddenly flying up in a Rockette high kick. The long-term result isn't funny at all. The smooth finish of cartilage in the joint has worn away, exposing the bone beneath. Now the bones of the ball and the socket are grinding against each other like the stones of a grist mill.

I have learned a lot about pain.

It has been recommended by several specialists that I have another surgery. Usually, they'd do a hip replacement, but the very spasms that caused the problem make this solution unworkable. Too much tension. Instead, they suggest that the ball at the top of my upper leg bone, my femur, be cut off.

The lead surgeon tells me that this is called the Girdlestone procedure. He says that it would end the grinding between the bones, and, he says, the pain. It would also mean that what was once a strong but mostly uncooperative leg would be rendered pretty much useless. The doctor says I shouldn't worry about that too much, though, because I can't really walk now, anyway. This makes me wonder if he ever considered a career as a diplomat. The road not taken, I guess.

I do not want this procedure, but pain is a powerful motivator.

On September 3, 2003, I hand out more Clooney pictures, and the ball of my right femur is surgically removed.

My parents come to the hospital, post-op. They wheel me to a lounge area where we can talk. Through the fog of medication, I try to allay their fears. "I'm fine," I say. But as they wheel me back to my room, they still seem worried, unconvinced. Then, turning to leave, my mom says, "Oh, my hat!" I tell her she'd left it on a gurney in the hall by the elevator. My parents laugh. I had glanced at her hat, had remembered it, and, despite the drug haze, had the presence of mind to connect the memory and my mom's words. I know, it's not exactly at the level of Sherlock Holmes, but my mom and dad seem to be reassured that I am going to be okay.

The post-surgical pain will linger for more than four years.

57

THROUGH A WIDE-ANGLE LENS

Becoming Comfortable in the Eye of the Camera

2007
The global financial house of cards is swaying now, about to collapse.
Sergei Polunin is named the Young British Dancer of the Year.

I MAY HAVE GIVEN THE impression that I was bedridden for years, recovering from one surgery after another, but it's not like that. In fact, with the help of friends, family, and the judicious use of painkillers, I have remained pretty active.

In the early days of my recovery from hip surgery, I turned my apartment into a performance space, complete with curtains and lighting. Calling it "Barefoot Theater," I would send invitations to all my friends who were dancers, actors, poets, and performance artists, sometimes suggesting a theme. One day we created a cooking show. Each guest showed up as a different outrageous chef and prepared some exotic dish. It ended in a feast. Over time, the pain subsided, but I kept the theater going for several years due to popular demand. Hosting a theater salon beats cable any day.

Remy Charlip would regularly light up the stage at the "Barefoot Theater" until 2005, when he had a pretty serious stroke. The children's book he wrote before the stroke, *A Perfect Day*, just came out. He recently sat for the drawings of the title character in the book *The Invention of Hugo Cabret*. Remy asked me if I could finish his next book for him. It's called *Dance Anywhere*. I told him that I didn't think I could do it, but he told me, "Of course, you can!"

I started getting out more. I once again joined the Gay Pride Parade in San Francisco. I've always felt a sense of solidarity with gay people. I've struggled with issues of self-pride, hiding myself in my cloak of invisibility. I've also struggled with people labeling me and making me feel uncomfortable about sex. The gay pride movement addresses all of that, from a slightly different vantage point, sure, but there's a similarity. And they are being quite in-your-face about it. Very bold. I admire the way they reclaimed the word "queer." Just took it back. Here, in this small contingent of people using wheelchairs, rolling down Market Street in San Francisco, I feel very welcomed by gay people, very understood. And their culture inspires me, I draw strength from it. Maybe disabled people can reclaim some words. Like "spastic." This parade encourages me to believe that disabled culture can become as powerful a force in society as gay culture. I believe that just being here helps to make that happen.

The old Sears building in San Francisco has been turned into an artists' colony of sorts, filled with stages and studios. For years, a dancer who lives there, Bob Webb, has hosted an event called "Bare Bones *Butoh*," where practitioners of the art, including the Tamanos, gather to perform. I've been on the program several times. But even when I'm not on the program, I go on stage during the intermission, performing my heart out. I'm not as mobile as I was before the hip surgery. I sort of drag my right leg when I stand up now, keeping my balance by leaning on something or someone. But

I dance in my chair and on the floor without inhibition. No one minds. They love watching. I take the stage.

And, at 53 years old, I've become a model.

~

I'm in a photographer's studio, sitting on a black floor, against a black background.

In front of the camera, facing the bright studio lights.

"Ready, Neil?"

"Yeah."

Here comes the camera.

When I first became disabled, I couldn't even look people in the eye, never mind look into the lens of a camera. Why not? Because I feared I was ugly. I thought that if I looked someone right in the eye, they would see me. See the monster.

I still remember the torture of the annual school pictures. Caught in the spotlight. No escape. Exposed for all to see. Captured on film.

As the camera starts clicking and whirring, I think about human beauty and how it is defined.

So much of the focus in our culture is on the body. And so many people are unhappy with their bodies. For many, this focus has become an obsession that elbows aside any consideration of the human spirit.

It seems to me that a sort of cult has grown up around this obsession. Imagine all the gyms and beauty salons as places of worship. It isn't hard to do. Imagine the incessant ads for cosmetics, hair treatments, and weight loss miracles as sermons, as homilies. It's easy if you try. Imagine cosmetic surgery, with its boob jobs, tummy tucks, and liposuction as a form of ritual scarring and sacrifice. Imagine all the people in fashion shows and beauty pageants as participants in sacred ceremonies.

And what is the reward being dangled in front of all these zealous cult members? What salvation, just out of reach? Nothing less than beauty as revealed in the holy scripture, *Vogue* and *GQ*.

To be fair, though, when a cult gets big enough, it has to be called a religion. A handful of disciples may be a cult, but a million faithful? That's a religion. And there are far more members in this cult than there are Episcopalians. So, what we're really talking about here is the Church of the Body. It may just be the biggest religion in the world. Maybe someday you'll join it.

The Church of the Body may not be a good fit for me. According to its dogma, I am damned. I am a misshapen rogue lamb who has to be culled from the flock. The Church warns that to look for beauty in bodies that don't conform to the scripture's strict standards is heresy.

So. I am the heretic who teaches that beauty has little to do with abs, implants, or nose jobs. I am the non-believer who must be barred from the temple.

Great. It's time to redefine beauty. What do I have to lose?

Nothing.

Now, I go for it. Straight into the camera. There's nothing to hide.

As Muhammad Ali said, "I am beautiful."

My face is unpredictable. All kinds of expressions just pop up whenever, wherever. Involuntarily. My jaw drops. My nostrils flare. My eyebrows soar. Anything. Beyond my control. I used to want to hide these random facial expressions. But now I look at it differently. I call it "acting."

Here he is, a cheeky disabled person, acting outrageously in public. Out there. Without inhibition. Defying expectations. Without shame. And no one knows what he'll do next, or what facial expression he'll come up with next. Okay, maybe it's a cheap shot, but it's sure been working for me. And it seems to be a revolutionary idea.

My mission now is to cultivate being a spastic, to develop the role. To embrace my inner and outer spaz. To play with extreme labored speech. To use people's curiosity and astonishment like any good performer does. In this new paradigm, my body itself becomes the medium in a new and shocking art form. A disabled body defined in artistic terms. People seem to be willing to give this new art form a chance, but for it to work, I have to believe in it.

Art. Performance. Disability. Body. This is my mantra to foster belief.

Disability is an art.

I am art.

These days, I find it great fun to play in front of the camera, to play with the camera. Most people fear it, but to me, it is my art. The challenge is to relax, in body and mind, so that I can simply be who I am in front of the camera. I maintain that being who you are isn't really all that simple. Maybe being who you are is the most challenging pose of all. Try it and you'll see.

~

The lights just went out.

"Damn it. Five minutes, Neil."

"Okay."

The photographer leaves.

As I sit in the dark, waiting for the lighting to be fixed, I think about fear and disability. I remember the self-perpetuating feedback loop of fear I first thought of in my shack back in Mankas. The loop that everyone, disabled or not, seems to be trapped in. Fear going back and forth, feeding on itself.

I think I understand it better now.

The way I see it, back in the Dark Ages, people believed in all kinds of preposterous nonsense. Magic, demons, monsters, vampires. Today, however, people put their faith in science, reason, logic, and rationality. We now believe that the laws of physics govern this world. We no longer believe in nonsense.

But.

There is another side to the modern mind. Its projections are on millions of flickering screens. What's on those screens? Magic, demons, monsters, and vampires. And, of course, endless violence and pornography. Do these images look like the products of a rational mind? No. But we love these images. Just look at the box office.

When we sailed out of the Dark Ages, the darkness sailed with us, stowed away below deck.

I recently saw a movie in which a slimy alien pops out of John Hurt's chest and kills everyone except Sigourney Weaver. This movie was made by and for the part of the brain that runs screaming from goblins, not the part that does crossword puzzles.

Each of us has an innate system that constantly looks for threats to survival, whether a growling dog, a runaway truck, or a hooded gunman. And when a threat is detected, a switch is automatically thrown that causes the heart to pound, the breath to quicken, and a dozen other changes in body and mind that prepare us to either fight or run for our lives. This is the fear response. This system has been hammered out by evolution over millions of years to help us survive.

Does it work?

Well, here we are.

But how does this system quickly and reliably sort through all the potential threats that this world can pose? It doesn't. It can't. It's much simpler than that. Think of two possible settings. If the system were set to throw the fear switch too readily, a lot of energy and time would be wasted responding to false alarms. If, on the other hand, the system were set to throw the fear switch only in extremis, at the point of death, then false alarms would not be the problem, death would. In other words, if real threats can sneak undetected past your system's perimeter and the fear switch is never thrown, well, you die. And, generally speaking, people who waste time responding to false alarms tend to have more children than people who are dead.

I'm pretty sure this is how evolution fashioned a human fear switch that is so easily tripped. The primitive default setting follows a simple rule:

It is better to be safe than sorry.

So. Almost anything that has the remotest chance of threatening survival can set it off. Even watching a movie that shows an alien slaughtering a spaceship's crew can make your heart pound.

That may explain why the fear switch is set to be so easily tripped, but how does the system determine whether something is a threat in the first place?

I think the answer is simple. Difference.

The system reacts to differences in potential threats. Here, small differences automatically make potential threats real. Which differences affect you is largely determined by the environment in which you were born and raised. A city kid, for example, may fail to read the warning signs that a bull is about to charge. He may blithely continue taking selfies. A country kid may not know how to read and safely navigate a downtown sidewalk.

Sometimes people look at me and they don't see me. I can see it in their eyes, in their faces, in their body language. They look at me, see my difference, then, in a flash, before rationality can intercede, deep in the most reptilian part of their brains, the fear switch is thrown. As though they have seen the alien that bursts out of John Hurt's chest. And the threat alarm sounds. Disgust. Horror. Fear. The call goes out.

"Monster! Monster! Monster!"

It is, of course, a false alarm. I am not a freak, not a monster. Much time and energy will be wasted in responding to the threat that I am mistakenly seen to be. But the instruction encoded in the genes and activated by the environment has been followed. In evolutionary terms, these people that I have horrified will be free to go forth and multiply. To pass the fear baton on to the next generation.

It looks like the photographer has finished. He just came back in.

The good news is that something that is a daily and pleasant part of a child's world is unlikely to be categorized later as a threat, or as a difference that throws the switch of fear. After all, kids raised with disabled siblings don't usually fear them. What would happen if disability became an integral and pleasant part of the daily lives of children everywhere? Imagine positive images of disability flickering on those millions of screens. On every TV, in every theater. Forget the movie *Alien*. I'm optimistic that the right environment can strengthen the part of the mind that tames fear. The rational and good part of the mind can be put in charge. In the driver's seat.

The house lights come on. It must have been a fuse. The photographer is fiddling with the lighting levels now.

"You okay, Neil?"

"Yeah."

"Okay. Almost ready."

While we are living in the final days of the Dark Ages of disability, there are still people who believe in monsters. The only monsters around here are either fictitious, like the one in *Alien,* or imaginary, like the one that some people with unfortunate childhoods see when they look at me. That monster lives only in their minds.

I guess you could say that in the world of disability we are living at the dawn of the Enlightenment, at the start of a new phase in the evolution of human society. Well, it can't come soon enough for me.

⁓

The studio lighting is on now. I'm sitting on a black floor, against black background. I turn toward the camera and look through it at the person who will look at this picture. Right in the eye.

"Okay. Neil, now turn your head a little to the right."

"Okay."

"No, your right."

58
ALLIES
Cultivating My Academic Side

2008

Michael Phelps swims his way to eight gold medals
at the Beijing Olympics.
Barack Obama wins the presidency.

I'M STILL IN BERKELEY. My mom died. My sister Wendy's here, helping out.

While I've been keeping pretty busy since my latest round of surgeries, I haven't had to turn down offers to star in Broadway plays, Hollywood movies, or prime-time network series. The hard truth is that there still aren't that many major roles written for tongue-tied spastics in wheelchairs. Mostly, I've been moping around the house between photo shoots, nursing a very painful hip. And not feeling very hopeful.

I still want to help build disability culture but am not sure how I can best be of service.

I prefer a play to a seminar, the stage to the lecture hall, but for disability culture to really take root and spread like kudzu, disabled people have to be everywhere in it, not just on the stage. Of course, we need disabled writers, directors, and editors to create and shape new works. But we also need disabled hair stylists, make-up artists, and costume designers to bring them to life. We even need disabled critics to misinterpret and viciously attack the works, to deconstruct the masterpieces of this new culture. There must also be disabled philosophers, historians, and sociologists to help reveal the truth, shape the narrative, and clear the path. And we certainly need clear-eyed disabled professors laboring in the ivy-covered halls, opening young minds to this cultural transformation, tuning them to this new wavelength. A thriving disability culture needs more than just a few spastics in the spotlight. We must be ubiquitous.

Think of it this way. It wasn't enough to secure the beachhead at Normandy, the hinterland had to be liberated, too. And the camps. For a job that big, you need an entire army. This calls for a recruitment drive.

I've acquired a certain reputation in the academic community. My plays, poetry, essays, and interviews are now often cited or reprinted in textbooks, anthologies, and scholarly journals. Images from my performances pop up in disability literature all the time. *Storm Reading* was broadcast on PBS and has become a fixture in Disabled Studies classes around the world. More and more, I see my work on the internet. Guest lecturing occasionally at Berkeley hasn't hurt my credibility, either. I seem to have been cast as a sort of "bad boy" of disability culture. Striking poses, strutting a little. As you know, I wanted the part. Well, I got it. I seem to be a quasi-punk spastic actor, poet, and multi-media artist. Academia has taken notice of me.

I just got an invitation to attend a symposium at the University of Michigan in Ann Arbor, as a poet and performance artist. I'd like to go, but it would just be too hard. All the travel, all the logistical difficulties. All the pain. I emailed my regrets.

Within hours, Dr. Petra Kuppers called me. She's the professor who is organizing the symposium. It's about the similarities between Black and disability cultures. She told me that they could pay for a helper for me, that they would pay for everything. They'd even pay for Wendy to come. She said that she really wanted me to come. She talked me into it.

∼

Dr. Kuppers meets us at the airport in Ann Arbor. She is elegantly dressed, using crutches, taller than me. Her clothes seem to drape and flow with her. "Call me Petra."

We talk as she drives us to the hotel, passing through frozen fields under gray skies. She is a disabled tenured professor at a major university. She owns her own home and remodels it however she wants. She is a feminist. She has taken complete charge of her life. Hearing about how she lives her life forces me to see that I am still dependent on my family. I begin to see her as a role model for me, and a kind of authority figure.

In the afternoon, Petra joins me in the hotel pool. Outside the window, it looks like Antarctica. Inside, Petra and I are floating in a steaming zero-gravity dance hall, while Wendy films us, hovering protectively. Petra, it turns out, is a strong swimmer, more at home in the water than on land, because of her back. She is like a sleek otter.

At the symposium, during the lunch break, Petra tells me, "You have been infantilized, Neil. You are being treated like a child." Petra pulls no punches.

She tells me I am an adult now, 54 years old, and I must make my own decisions about my life and stop relying on my parents, and my brothers and sisters. She makes me think a lot about what I really want in my life. I realize that I want to belong somewhere. I want it to be perfectly natural for me to be there and to be equal, to be valued. I need privacy, and autonomy. I crave these things. To me, Petra represents independence.

A home. A warm welcome. Freedom.

Petra was born in Germany in the late 60s. She says that when she was little, she developed problems with her back and legs and a specialist told her that she would never perform on stage. She says that instead of meekly slipping into the mental restraints he was holding out for her to try on, instead of accepting his invitation to start down the long dark and limiting road of self-pity, she became defiant, even a little angry, and then, with great style, added "performer" to her list of life goals. Now she is known as the multi-disciplinary professor who writes, lectures, directs, and performs on stage in her wheelchair.

One of her creations is the Olimpias Project, a consortium of artists, performers, and academics that produces books, plays, films, and multi-media events that explore human differences and cultivate disability culture. One part of it is the Helping Dance Group. Participants are encouraged to utilize the dancers to get the help they want. I attended today and asked for help standing and hugging. Petra recently had a gallery show of works generated by Olimpias: "The Myth of Difference." These artists are breaking new ground.

It is the second day, and Petra has started calling me "lovey" and "my dear" in her adorable German accent. Her attitude to relationships is quite open. I think of it as European. She's very direct about these matters. She tells me that I'm sexy. She laughs when I insist that I'm not, then tells me that denying it makes me even sexier. We seem to be hitting it off.

I think she recognizes the benefits that come with our shared knowledge of what it's like to be different. As different as our ways of expressing our visions are, she seems to have decided that we are on the same mission. I think she's right. We quickly feel a close kinship.

As we say our goodbyes at the airport, Petra invites me to visit her during the summer break, when she won't be so busy.

～

The first thing Petra told me when I arrived back in Ann Arbor was that when she first met me, she thought I was a Lothario. The fields we were driving through had turned lush and green.

"What's a Lothario?" I asked.

"I thought you were a lady-killer," she said, laughing. "He was one of Shakespeare's inventions, in *Othello*."

"That's not me," I insisted.

She laughed louder and said, "Neil, that's exactly what a Lothario would say!"

We make an odd couple, I think. There are some stark contrasts. For example, once people tame their fear of disability, they usually find me likable. Not so with Petra. She can be brusque once in a while. Sometimes twice. While I am fairly small, she is not. While I'm famous, particularly in Petra's social and academic circles, I am usually quite humble about it. That is not her style. More than anything else, she tells me, she wants security. I tell her, "So do I!" We are a perfect match.

We are filmed dancing on the floor together for a movie called *Tiresias*, completely covered by a red silk sheet. Beneath it, we are naked and I give her a kiss, all unseen by crew and audience. The kiss wasn't in the script. I did it impulsively. She immediately tells all of her friends about it.

～

It is August now, and Petra has come to Berkeley for the Disability Film Festival. She stays with me.

In the theater, we enjoy each other much more than the films.

She starts using her frequent flyer miles to visit me on weekends. She rents a van with a lift, so we can go anywhere we want. Before you know it, she is living with me three days a week. Then I start using my frequent flyer miles, commuting between California and Michigan. Soon, we are together more than we're apart.

I am growing more confident, more autonomous.

In December, I make a decision.

"Wendy. I. Think. You. Can. Go. Now. I'll. Be. Okay." This is a big deal for me.

Wendy says, "I'll start looking for a place." She moves to Arcata, up north.

A little problem pops up between my dad and Petra. My dad seems to think that Petra isn't good for me. Maybe he thinks her influence is making me too independent. I'm not sure. Petra tells me that my dad told her that she should start paying rent. She answered him.

"Nein."

I'm not really worried about it. Petra can handle him.

When I am with Petra, I have the feeling that I am really free.

We start working together, building disability culture.

Collaborating.

Traveling.

Loving.

59
SEDUCTION WITH IDEAS
We Nurture Disability Culture

Early 2011

In February, IBM's artificially intelligent computer, Watson, outsmarts
the humans on Jeopardy.

The Oscar for Best Picture goes to *The King's Speech*.

The Smithsonian's website features the works of Neil Marcus.

~

FOR THE PAST FEW YEARS, Petra and I have been taking our show on the
road, traveling around the country together. She tells me about the ideas
of the philosopher Michel Foucault, who sees society as a hierarchy of
power relationships created and held in place by the control of language,
its knowledge, categories, and expectations. There is an arbitrariness to this
view that I find hopeful. It suggests that such things aren't innate or fixed. It
suggests that it can all be changed. The relationships, the expectations, the
society itself.

I could say that we are like the apostles, spreading the gospel, but it's
not like that. The comparison that I like best is John Chapman, who spent

sixty years wandering up and down the Ohio Valley planting small apple orchards. His whole life was dedicated to planting seeds. He is remembered as Johnny Appleseed.

Petra makes the arrangements with the hosting organizations and handles all the logistics for flights and hotels. She is very organized. Amazing, in fact.

When it's showtime, Petra is the ringmaster. She and I sit at the front in our chairs. She begins, talking softly, relaxing the audience with her soothing voice, assuring them that all is well and all will be well. Slowing them down. Setting the tone.

Then she talks about the differences between people and how these differences have been dealt with by society historically, how they are dealt with today. She has the group do a few relaxing and centering exercises, to get them to give themselves some space, some time. I've heard her call what she does "modulating people's energies."

Using a big screen behind us, she introduces material sent by people who aren't in the room. Some of these contributors attend virtually, eyes glued to screens in other states, in other countries. Some of them participate in real time. They read poetry. Tell stories. Show short films. Sing snippets from operas. Quote diction. fantasy. biography.

The people who are actually in the room participate as well. Some of the program is prearranged, some spontaneous. We hear more life stories . Petra gently guides each session, from start to finish, presenting the contributions of people from all over, drawing on the life experiences and creativity of all the participants, weaving together dance, songs, films, pictures, stories, and poetry, connecting it all with an improvised but focused narrative. She weaves a beautiful tapestry.

And what is my role? I keep my finger on the pulse of the group. I monitor their mood, their anxiety, curiosity, and receptiveness. Gauge laughter. Assess body language. Listen to emotional overtones in voices. And then, when I sense an opening, a moment when the group is ready to accept something new, I stand on my left leg, leaning against my chair or against Petra in hers, and slowly deliver the handful of words that I have chosen for that precise moment. I try to use no more than 17 syllables at a time, similar to haiku. Any more than that and I've found the message takes too long, losing the strength found in brevity.

For example, here we are in Michigan, in a room of forty people, most of them seated on the floor.

I speak. "Take. Off. Your. Shoes."

In a soft voice, Petra repeats my message, adding, "Only if you want to."

"Lean. On. Each. Other."

This time she adds, "Make sure you have permission. Make sure it's okay."

"No. Lean. More. Harder."

She adds, "Make sure you have their consent."

"We. Are. Like. Water. Fluid."

Petra just repeats this. No additions.

"This. Is. Love." No additions.

"To. Sum. It. All. Up. Bare. Feet. Touch. Support. Water. Fluidity. Love. That's. All."

And, as I speak, I dance, I share my body and my self with the group, showing them that my way of being in the world is very different than most people's. And, as I dance and speak, I touch Petra on her shoulders, her arms, her head. I demonstrate the importance of touch, of contact, of dance.

Even if I were to say nothing, the message I send by simply being here is delivered, and received. This is disability. There is nothing to fear. This is beauty. This is art. Do not feel threatened. There is no threat. Relax. Feel free. Feel love.

The message can be a little shocking: Two disabled people, up here, up front. Publicly displaying affection. And attraction. I am very careful not to go too far with participants, not to make them too uncomfortable. I don't want them to shut down or freak out. And I can tell when they feel it, when they get it. I know the moment when they feel freed.

The underlying themes of the program are always the same.

Liberate. End oppression.

Integrate. End isolation.

Connect. Empower. Mobilize. End the lack of touch, access, and mobility.

Free. End institutionalization.

Humanize. End revictimization.

And the overarching message that informs all the others: disability is a beautiful thing, an enriching presence in the world. Properly conceived, disability is an art. It is an ingenious way to live in this world. Disability heightens and deepens people's understanding of freedom, and, more importantly, of love.

When we travel, we try to stay in hotels with swimming pools. In a second-hand store in Berkeley, I found an old Kodak underwater camera. I bought it for 35 dollars. We tried it out in a pool in Berkeley. It's not state-of-the-art, but it works great.

Petra and I talk it over and decide to hold part of our sessions outside the lecture hall. Everyone into the pool!

The change from air to water, from one gravity to zero gravity, from clothing to bathing gear, alters the whole dynamic of the group. The possibilities of movement, touch, and dance multiply as people with different abilities interact in the pool. We interact in ways that just aren't possible on dry land. We fly in liquid. We film the results, randomly, letting chance be the photographer. I select and edit the best shots, which are then projected on the big screen behind us back in the meeting room.

What should we call these sessions? They aren't lectures. Not movies or plays. Not concerts. They're not really workshops, either. They certainly aren't dances or pool parties. Not exclusively, anyway. The boundaries are gone. The defining lines are blurred. We decide to call them salamanders, after the amphibian that alchemists believe was born in fire.

Our salamanders open doors for me and for disability culture. We are pioneers, trekking up the Archangel Valley of culture, sowing seeds as we go.

It is fun to travel and see so many places.

We even get to see the far side of the world.

60

KANGAROO HEAVEN

Experts in Australia

Late 2011

Scientists prove that Australian Aborigines migrated out of Africa

60,000 years ago.

The book *Cripple Poetics* comes out, too. Petra and I wrote the poems

together. A journal of our courtship.

I'M ON AN ISLAND OFF the south coast of Australia. I'm in my chair on its southern shore, facing the sea. Straight ahead of me, across 4,600 miles of open ocean, is Antarctica. I'm 57, and I'm farther away from home than I've ever been.

Petra and I have been in Australia for weeks now. We're here at the invitation of the Australian government, to consult on disability culture. We've been all over. The people here are happier than the people back home. One thing they say a lot is "no worries." I think they mean it.

A lot of the older people here make this certain gesture when they see me. It goes like this. Click your tongue through your teeth out the side of your mouth. At the same time, wink and quickly cock your head. Make sure your eyes are smiling. The unspoken message is something like, "Ah, yes, I remember the war," or "God love ya," or "Poor bastard." In fact, I think it's a mixture of all three. In about equal parts.

In Sydney, we went to a concert starring Archie Roach. He sang "Took the Children Away." It's about the Australian government's old policy of taking Aboriginal babies away from their mothers and giving them to white families. Archie was one of those babies.

We attended a memorial for the disabilities activist Christopher Newell at the University of New South Wales in Sydney. He taught there. He was sort of like the Ed Roberts of Australia. The memorial was held in a hall that looked and felt like it was in the British Houses of Parliament.

Petra and I were there as guest poets. My allotted time on the panel was five minutes. I was wearing a bright red shirt that had been presented to me about a year ago during a ceremony at a pow-wow in California. When my turn came, I stood up and slowly took off my pow-wow shirt. Then I slowly put on a yellow t-shirt emblazoned with the slogan, "Disability is an Art." I let the message marinate for a moment, then launched into a labored but resonant version of "Somewhere Over the Rainbow." Judging by the smiles, the song went over well.

During a workshop, a young woman named Kelly had something to say.

"Who was the wally with the broight idea to push a puhson in a wheelcheah out onto a stage and make them lip-synch to Celine bloody Dion and dance with Big Buhd? That's not aht. And it's not roight. It's humiliating and it has to stop. I want betta. I demand betta!"

Too right, Kelly. If all we accomplished by traveling more than half-way to the South Pole was to provide backup for people like you, it would have been a worthwhile trip.

∽

While I am somewhat creative, in most practical matters, I am inept. I think Petra got tired of waiting for me to act decisively. Her way was to go for it. Come on! Make a plan! Do it!

In the end, she moved on with someone else. I don't blame her.

I said, "Okay, I'll join in the breakup." It hurt though.

Those eight years together were astounding. What fun it was! But she left.

61

I'm About to Be Wedded

I Grapple with Love Again

Early 2016
It looks like the Republican Party may nominate Donald Trump.
They find water on Mars.

~

REMY PASSED AWAY. Ben Kingsley played the title role in Scorsese's film *Hugo*.

My dad died.

Mark O'Brien's article "On Seeing a Sex Surrogate" was adapted to the screen as *The Sessions*. Helen Hunt was nominated Best Supporting Actress for her portrayal of the surrogate.

A surgeon replaced the bones of my left shoulder joint with pieces of sculpted plastic. He couldn't do the right shoulder because the muscle spasms on that side would have pulled all the plastic pieces apart.

Wendy's gone. My new assistant, Anna, moved into the spare room. Everyone I know seems to be moving now. Like musical chairs.

Anna helped me with the rehab from my shoulder surgery. At first, I would wake up in the middle of the night screaming in pain, my arms frozen, my body wracked with multiple spasms. She would come in and help me unlock my arms.

Berkeley recently legalized marijuana for medical use. My doctor was pretty sure that it would help me and wrote me a prescription, but the doe-eyed clerk down at the medical marijuana dispensary didn't even want to see it. She took one look at me and handed me a big bag of weed. When I offered her some money, she waved her delicate hand, palm out, saying, "Nah, man, it's all good." That may not seem like much, but I consider such small gestures to be one of the little perks of disability. And, oh, the doctor was right.

Anna came here a few years ago from Ukraine. A blue-eyed, honey blonde with a warm smile and an endearing accent, she's in her early forties. I'm 63, so that means she's young to me. I need more help than I once did with bathing, dressing, and hygiene. She helps with my pain meds, with my daily life. She's really good at it, and I don't mean that she's just good at the various tasks involved, I'm talking about the attitude that she brings to the job.

Let's face it, not all of the people who serve as caregivers love their work. Some do it because they can't find a better job. Their pay is about the same as a teaching assistant. Such people may do their assigned tasks well, but their attitude is sometimes one of resignation, or worse, resentment. I can usually spot it right away. It's in the tone of voice. There's a sort of artificial camaraderie, and a fake buoyancy. Also, when they're doing a job, like helping me get dressed, there's this almost robotic competency. And it's not like they're trying to fool me so much as they're trying to fool themselves. If you've never needed help like this, you probably don't understand how important it is that the person helping you isn't doing it grudgingly. I don't really blame them. Life is rough.

There is nothing inherent about the job that makes it an ordeal, though. It depends on how you approach it. And Anna has figured that out. She enjoys her work. She tells jokes. I tell jokes. We have fun together. We laugh. Anna really likes being with me. And I like being with her. She even stars in little films we make together. Children's stories, mostly. Stuff we write. Goofy stuff. We both laugh as we make them. On camera, off camera. We are giddy. Having giggle fits.

Is there a line that you step over when you fall in love? One side, not love; the other, love? A biochemical border that must be crossed, an emotional passport that must be stamped? Maybe. I'm not sure. But if there is such a border, I'm pretty sure I have inadvertently wandered over it. Unknowingly stumbled across the frontier.

Let's see. Yup. No doubt about it. I'm in love.

And guess what. I think she loves me, too.

When we talk now, we gaze at each other, all smiles. In her eyes, I see great wisdom, passed down through centuries. I also feel great warmth. I see Anna's eyes filled with love for me. I am intoxicated.

Our talk turns to the future. We are already happily living together. We are in love. And the subject is broached. I brought it up. We talk about marriage. About being together forever. She laughs and smiles. She says we could live happily ever after.

Wow. I am stunned. Me. Happily married. Us. Together forever.

It's Sunday. Anna is out and my friend Daniel drops by, instantly making the apartment feel small.

We sit together in my living room. Facing each other. Chair to chair.

"Anna. And. I. Are. In. Love," I say. I watch his reaction carefully.

"That's great, Neil! Congratulations, man!" says Daniel, his voice filling my apartment.

I cut to the chase. "I. Think. She. Wants. Us. To. Get. Married."

"Dude! That's a big step," says Daniel, but not in a cautionary way. It sounds more like glee.

"What. Should. I. Do?" I honestly want his opinion. He is more worldly than me. More seasoned.

He tugs his beard twice. His pate shines. His eyes glisten. "Go for it, Neil!"

A few days later, I get down on one knee in front of Anna. I take out the ring I bought and hold it out to her.

"Anna. Will. You. Marry. Me?"

⁓

That was months ago. I would like to explain exactly what happened after I proposed to Anna.

But I can't.

A while ago, my doctor told me to ease up on my use of painkillers. It is not as easy as it sounds. I seem to have acquired a bit of a habit. But I'm tough, I can do this. So I cut back and, there it is, the familiar pain of osteoarthritis. In my shoulder, my wrist, my neck.

Then, as I slowly break the habit, a mental fog lifts. I can see things more clearly. It's very strange. I hadn't even realized that I was in a fog. My thoughts become sharper, with more perspective. Now, looking back, my romance with Anna is like a half-forgotten dream.

I was really socked in.

I remember clearly that she didn't answer the question, "Will you marry me?" with the word "no." In fact, at the time, I thought she seemed delighted. Looking back, it may be that she was amused, or maybe just nervous, or uncomfortable. My intuition may have misfired.

In any case, I thought I'd heard a "yes" and began to make wedding plans.

I went to Kendra's house in the hills above Berkeley. Unlike Daniel, she urged caution. She suggested that we visit an attorney for advice. I knew she was just trying to protect her baby brother, but I thought of her divorce and wondered if she could really be objective. Down through the years, though, I have learned that when I need unbiased and unvarnished advice, Kendra is always there, smart and very practical. Anyway, I agreed to go.

I can't remember everything the lawyer said, but the gist of it was that marrying Anna would be problematic. We could get married, but then we would have to convince the government that we were really in a relationship. The fact that she was my caregiver and more than 20 years younger than me would make that harder, he said. The government would ask for proof that she wasn't marrying me just to stay in the country. That would be fraud, he said. He also told us that she wouldn't be able to sponsor her daughter who, at 22, was simply too old. Lenny explained about the finances, too. Anna's sponsor had to have a job. I'd have to prove I had enough income to keep Anna off welfare. All my assets might have to be shared with her, if she became my ex.

While I didn't think this bleak scenario was very likely, I do remember thinking that I didn't really want to have to start playing musical chairs.

Together, Kendra and I presented what we learned to Anna. Kendra did most of the talking. The presentation wasn't blunt, but neither was it exactly gentle. Kendra put the raw information on the table, without drawing conclusions. For example, she did not say that we should not get married. She did, however, list all the hurdles and pitfalls that the lawyer had told us about.

I thought that Anna took it all very well. She didn't ask many questions, didn't really say much at all. Her expression was that of someone who was interested in what was being said, but not surprised by it, and certainly not worried about it. When Kendra was finished, Anna smiled and thanked her for her help in looking into these matters. I remember thinking as I looked at my fiancée's face that we were going to go through with it. I thought that, together, we were going to surmount all the hurdles. As Kendra headed to the elevator, I heard wedding bells, thinking, "Mr. and Mrs. Marcus." I felt sure that we were going to get married.

If I remember it right, it was the next day that I began to notice little things about Anna that I had not noticed before. The first one that comes to mind is her telling me to sit up straight when I was eating. I don't think that she had ever said that to me before. Not long after that, she showed concern about the tidiness of my breakfast tray. That was a new one, too. I'm pretty sure it was, anyway. As the days passed, I thought that I was beginning to detect a note of criticism in much of what she said, as though an underlying impatience was coloring every word. I remember thinking that she was almost snapping at me.

Why?

I don't know for sure, but I've been thinking about it and have a few theories.

I may have misread what was merely a flirtation as something much more, and Anna was adopting this new persona to correct my misunderstanding. Gently backing me away from a romance that only existed in my imagination.

Anna may have been hoping to solve her immigration problems through matrimony, and Kendra's little talk had throttled this hope in its cradle. Her seemingly sudden interest in the arrangement of the remains of my scrambled eggs could have been her way of signaling to me that the foundation of our engagement had just collapsed. Metaphorically speaking.

Or let's say Anna really had loved me, and Kendra's words, apparently delivered with my tacit blessing, were so insulting that her love for me died then and there. She may have thought that she was being accused of being selfish and cunning, even greedy. And it may be that when Anna helps someone she doesn't love, she channels Emily Post.

Or maybe it was me getting cold feet. Facing the prospect of spending the rest of one's life with someone else can focus the mind. As you approach the altar, tiny flaws once easily overlooked can be magnified by the imagination. Maybe Anna had always been a bit of a prissy nitpicker, and I just hadn't noticed.

I remember the growing feeling that I was in the first days of a life sentence of daily court-ordered etiquette classes. It sounds weird, but I had this glimpse of my future, sitting at breakfast, day after day, year after year, a round piece of cold sausage link on the end of a fork, hovering impatiently, a few inches from my mouth. The same greasy piece, every morning. In my vision, I look up and lock eyes with the person holding the fork. It is Anna, dressed as Nurse Ratched.

I arranged a meeting around my dinner table. Anna and her brother were there, as was my friend and neighbor, Raj, who's also a lawyer. My helper Patrick was there, too, and Kendra, of course. My plan was to clear the air, to talk things out, to give everyone a chance to air their grievances, to put their cards on the table. I remember harboring the hope that our engagement could be put right if only we could really communicate, heart to heart.

Anna acted surprised. She did not think the air needed clearing. She could not think of anything that needed to be talked out. She had no grievances, and no cards to put on the table. She was puzzled at the suggestion that she had become less patient. She asked Kendra to explain what "snapping" meant.

I started crying. I couldn't help it. At first, it was only tears, but soon I was sobbing. At the table with five other people, an old man in a wheelchair, crying his eyes out. Well, what would you do if what you were sure was your only hope for love and happiness was suddenly shown to be a mirage?

We stumbled on together for about a week. She came to work. She did her job. Politely. Competently.

Don't get me wrong. I loved Anna. I still do. But it seemed to me that even if she had once loved me, she no longer did. At that point, it really didn't matter which theory was right. Each of them might have held a piece of the truth. No matter. It just wasn't working anymore. Not for me, not for her, not for us.

I wrote her a letter.

Dear Anna,

I regret to say that the job you're doing as my helper is not working out well for me. I feel tension and conflict. It may be that our personalities simply clash. In any case, I'll be looking for a new helper.

I would appreciate it if you would move out as soon as you can.

Thank you for all your help and care. Over the past year, we had many great times and lots of love. I will do all that I can to help you with your future.

Sincerely,
Neil

I gave her the letter and watched her as she read it. I braced myself for tears, but there weren't any. No anger, either. It's possible that she felt relief. I'm not sure. I couldn't tell. But I knew I was alone again, broken-hearted.

And, yes, a little relieved.

~

A lot of very smart medical researchers have been trying to figure out how to get the best results from the wires lodged deep in my brain. Based on their research, they make adjustments to the jolts of electricity zapping my brain cells. After months of trial-and-error, these adjustments have improved my speech a little. There doesn't seem to be any difference in the non-speech muscle groups, though, and my joints feel like they're getting rustier. Especially in my neck.

Do they even know what they're doing?

62
MIND FIELD

An Anguished Deconstruction

2018

The Cassini probe plunges into Saturn.
Daddy Yankee raps on "Despacito."

~

BACK IN ABOUT 1975, when I was at Moorpark, I got a letter from Berkeley's Center for Independent Living. They were introducing themselves to disabled people everywhere. It was signed by Judy Heumann. Here is proof, I thought, proof of the existence of a whole movement of disabled people, out there in the real world. Proof that there are heroes.

Moses and I drove up together to check it out. We pulled up in front of an old, four-story building with hundreds of feet of zig-zagging wheelchair ramps wrapping around it, retrofitted to make every room on every floor easily accessible. I'd seen a couple of wheelchair ramps before, but nothing like this.

Inside, we found a beehive of activity. These people were on a mission. And every single one of them was disabled. I was shocked. As I looked around, then as I was shown around, my shock turned into delight. A whole office, a whole building, an entire enterprise, being run by and for my people. I couldn't contain my growing smile. I quit trying. Ear to ear.

∼

Shortly after the Center for Independent Living was founded in Berkeley, a mural was painted on the concrete retaining wall of its parking area. It depicted the people who had helped turn the dream of that first CIL into a reality. The founders. It was like our Mt. Rushmore.

In 2012, when the CIL was moved to its new Ed Roberts Campus, the mural, about 8 feet tall and 75 feet long, was left behind. An effort was made to have the mural designated as an historical landmark, but it didn't pan out. It looked like the mural's days were numbered. Would Mt. Rushmore be demolished?

Into the breach leapt the artist who had painted the mural. Discretion demands that he be called Tompkins here. He offered to create a mural at the new campus, better than the original. This idea was applauded by both the CIL's Board of Directors and the developer of the old site, who said he would support the project to the tune of $15,000. It was agreed that Tompkins would paint a scaled-down version of the new mural before the Board gave its final approval. The University of California in Los Angeles even agreed to provide $1,500 to help pay for this prototype.

Then another problem raised its ugly little head. It seems Tompkins was a resident of People's Park. Yes, he was homeless. Back then, UCLA had a very strict policy of not advancing funds directly to people who curled up on park benches at night.

Once again, the prospects for a mural looked bleak. What is needed, said UCLA, is a responsible party to whom we can entrust this $1,500, someone who can ensure that it is used to achieve the goals and objectives spelled out in the grant.

As the smoke slowly cleared, you could see there, ready to do battle, the seated figure of the internationally acclaimed writer/actor/dancer/artist, Neil Marcus. Rod Lathim, who was working with them, had suggested my name to them as a responsible party.

That's how, at the age of 64, I became the manager of the grant. I would be responsible for the "implementation of all grant-funded activities." I took my responsibilities seriously. I went so far as to arrange weekly meetings with Tompkins. The plan was that we dine together at my place on Thursdays. He would report on his progress and I would give him the portion of the grant money that the weekly report seemed to warrant.

It all seemed so reasonable at the time.

Prior to these dinners, I had not known Tompkins well. To say hello, sure. As an artist, yes. But not well.

At our first dinner, I learned that his childhood was harsh. He told me his father didn't want to raise a wimp.

He perseverates. At each dinner he says, "I'm no wimp!" He says this three or four times.

I try to counsel him, to console him, even, but it is useless. He tells me he perforated his eardrums target-shooting at beer bottles in Death Valley. Just blew them out.

So while I can talk to him, he can't really hear me. And while I can listen to him, we can't communicate.

But he sure can talk.

⁓

All this summer, the wildfires surrounding the Bay Area have been fierce, turning the air foul and dimming the sun. Wood smoke is everywhere, tickling your throat and scratching your lungs.

Between two of the mural dinners, I have emergency brain surgery in San Francisco.

It seems a buried suture has been festering in my scalp for fifteen years.

For two days, I am once more a hospital patient, receiving antibiotics intravenously, being held for observation. I feel positively gutted. I am beyond weary.

I'm discharged on the hottest day of the year. The air stinks. My throat hurts. My van has conked out, so a van taxi is hired to take me home. Its AC is stuck on cold, and I only have a light jacket. The driver has chosen a loud, muscular piano rendition of "Amazing Grace" for us. In spite of all these trials, I try to cling to the thought that I am a lucky man. The driver notices the tears running down my cheeks and turns to look at me.

"Are you okay?" she asks, genuinely concerned.

Sometimes, when I am exhausted, I can speak very clearly. "Yes, I'm okay," I say, very clearly.

⌁

So. Here I sit. At dinner again with Tompkins. Just out of the hospital. My lungs burn. My recently wounded heart has not yet healed. I am still emotionally fragile. My joints ache. My limbs are weak. My energy is low. I am not good and not getting better.

I pour out my heart to Tompkins. I tell him all about the surgery.

"You're the best, Neil!" he enthuses, apropos of nothing, "We make a great team!"

I can think of no interpretation of the present context that provides this utterance with meaning.

He launches into a lengthy, implausible explanation of his charitable work with Nicaraguan orphans who have cleft palates. Something about presents being sent at Christmas.

A thought comes to me from the wings of the stage in my brain. Maybe this is karma. A simple balancing of the cosmic books. An old, forgotten debt from another lifetime that has come due at last. Even as I think it, I know this thought isn't true and it isn't fair to Tompkins to even think it.

Finally, under the weight of all the stress, I collapse. I am physically and emotionally exhausted.

I break down.

Tompkins doesn't sleep in the park now. He works in a cryonics facility, draining the bodily fluid from dead people and replacing it with a plasma-like liquid that acts as a sort of antifreeze. He puts the bodies in big cylinders filled with liquid nitrogen. They'll stay in there until scientists find a cure for whatever killed them. Then they'll be thawed out, revived, and cured. Probably not by Tompkins, but, maybe. Who knows? He sleeps in the storeroom at the cryonics facility.

The new mural is almost finished. Mt. Rushmore renewed.

63

UNBELIEVABLY TRUE

The Play Is the Thing

August 2018

Yesterday, I watched Childish Gambino in the music video
for "This is America." Madness.

I also saw Justify win the Triple Crown. He's going to be
retired now. Undefeated.

AFTER BREAKFAST, ROD Lathim called to say he wants to reprise *Storm
Reading* for one more show. He asked me if I was interested.

Am I interested? I inhale. I have serious doubts that I would even be
able to do it. I have been resting since my breakdown, but I still have a lot
of pain in my neck, shoulder, and wrist. I also feel tired almost all the time.
I look out the window at the Golden Gate, at the ocean beyond, and take a
deep breath. I set all my doubts aside. I exhale.

"Of. Course. I'm. Interested."

So, on September 21, 2018, thirty years after its premiere, *Storm Reading*
will return to the stage of the Lobero Theater. Matthew Ingersoll and

Kathryn Voice will join me in presenting six live scenes that will be complemented by a screening of several others that were filmed there in 1996. The event will be hosted by Anthony Edwards. I feel my energy level rise just thinking about it.

~

The VIP reception is held in the courtyard behind the theater just before the performance. Friends and theater people are there. It is really good to see them again.

"Hi, Neil!"

"Hi!"

I smile, shake hands, pose for pictures, and I am amazed. The thirty years since the premiere have gone by in the blink of an eye. I was really a nobody back then, and now the aristocracy of the American Riviera has gathered here to rub shoulders with me. I'm the toast of the town.

~

The house lights are still on.

Once again, I am sitting in the wings of the Lobero Theatre. Thirty years to the day after the premiere of *Storm Reading*, I'm back in the same spot. Exactly. I touch the flattened coin taped to the arm of my chair.

They know who I am here. I am Neil Marcus, the handicapped performer who got his start right here. They know what to expect and what is needed. The doors backstage have all been propped open. The dressing room doors have been removed. Everything is perfectly in place, no mysteries, no hassles. There is even a ring of orange traffic cones around my parking place.

As I wait, I reflect. So much is the same. So much has changed.

The society I was born into was not built with disabled people in mind.

All the ramps, railings, and grab bars. All the curb cuts, widened doors, and transit lifts. The signs in braille, the closed captioning, and the chirping crosswalks. The wider hallways, reserved parking spots, and mandated elevators. All the cavernous bathroom stalls and the mesmerizing ASL interpreters. All of this is new. I saw it happen. It didn't happen by itself. A thousand heroes made it happen. And for disabled people, this is a different world, a much bigger world. I'm not saying it's perfect, far from it. But it's definitely better. I have to continue this journey. I must learn new tactics. It's required!

"Two minutes, Neil." A voice behind me. I nod.

Here's the real progress: to pretend that disabled people are invisible is now considered to be simply rude. Or consider identity politics: I, Neil Marcus, am now an interspecies interdisciplinary specialist in communication. And soon, all this talk about "humanizing" disabled people will be viewed as an amusing relic of a backward time in human history. Society changes. It can open up. It is happening right now. We can evolve.

The house lights are turned off. I'm ready now. Fully charged. I touch the flattened penny on the arm of my chair.

I'm on.

∿

Under the cover of the darkness, I roll out to the front of center stage.

I stop at my mark.

The spotlight is switched on.

I hear the audience listening.

I deliver the opening line that I wrote decades ago.

People are watching me. They're watching me all the time. They're watching me even when they're pretending not to watch me. They're watching me to see how well I do this thing called human. Every dream I ever had came true. The person that I never thought I was or could be, I am.

A wave of applause washes over me. Around the glow of the spot, I see people getting to their feet, clapping.

At this moment, I am a human bridge, spanning centuries of ideas, notions, and customs. Crossing over all the borders.

I am an artist. Everything I do is a brushstroke. Every word. Every movement. Every gesture. My life is my medium. And the canvas that I am applying my brushstrokes to is life itself, with humanity in the foreground.

Curtain.

64
Who's Who
Semi-Autobiography

Spring 2019
A Chinese robot named Yutu-2 is poking around inside a crater
on the dark side of the moon.
Macedonia just changed its name. Now it's North Macedonia.

I'm 65 years old.

While the trip down to Santa Barbara was plagued by logistical hiccups, the trip back was a breeze. At a Burger King somewhere near Salinas, I bumped into a member of Rod's production crew who had been at the Lobero the night before.

"It's you," she said.

"Yes," I answered. "It's. Me."

"I can't believe it!" she said. "What are the odds?"

"It's. A. Sure. Thing," I answered.

I ordered for everyone. Cheeseburgers, vanilla shakes, onion rings.

Back in 1971, not long after arriving at Fairhaven College, I went over to the library on the Western Washington State College campus to check out the biographies of famous spastics. There were no such books in the library. None. Right then, at 17, I decided that someday I would write my life story.

Since then, I saved everything I wrote and everything written about me. I also saved every piece of video or audio that includes my image or voice. I stored this collection in my guest room closet, squirreled away in stacks of cardboard boxes. Now much of it is housed in the archives of the Bancroft Library at UC Berkeley and, while I still have a few boxes, almost all of it is now in my computer as well. I have everything needed to write my biography.

I tried to write the book myself, but it didn't work. After many false starts and failed collaborations, it became clear to me that to write a book I would need more than creativity.

Then, after the *Storm Reading* revival at the Lobero, a recently retired friend who'd heard about my project came up and said, "I'd like to help out."

I said, "Ha. Le. Lu. Yah."

A couple of weeks after I got back to Berkeley, we started writing. That we lived thousands of miles apart meant that all of our communication would be digital. We used Google Docs. Most of our talk was through the chat and comments bar to the right of the document itself. We also used emails, and, when there was someone on my end to help interpret, the phone. I would type questions and suggestions into the chat bar, with one finger, of course. It took time.

Generally, I would send him something from my archive, he would read it, and then ask me questions. He would often ask about sequence, because many of the items in the archive are undated, and authorship, because many of the items are unsigned. Sometimes he would ask me to clarify details and what was going on in my life at that time. I would send scripts, pictures, and articles as attachments to emails. When he felt that he knew enough about that topic and how I viewed it, he would write a rough draft. Then I would add comments to guide him in the rewrite. We both worked to ensure that the ideas and opinions expressed were mine, not his, and that the words used to express them were consistent with what I would have written if I could type faster. We sought to create a narrative voice that is clearly mine, but more easily understood than my dystonic barrier would usually allow.

Little by little. Write, rewrite, polish. Word by word. Add here, delete there. Line by line. Copy, cut, paste. Page by page. Day by day. Chapter by chapter.

I am quite earnest about the writing of this book. I am inspired.

65
ONCE REMOVED

Stuck in Transit

Summer 2019
Notre-Dame, gutted by fire, will be rebuilt just as it was.
On the Swiss Hit Parade, the number one single is "Old Town Road."

ON AN UNUSUALLY HOT day in the spring, after a busy trip across the Bay, I was so exhausted that I fell to the floor by the toilet. Incredibly, my head got wedged under the toilet. Right away, the small but busy switchboard that regularly receives complaints from the various departments of my body rang headquarters to report that the two neck bones that had been screwed together years before were not amused by the whole "fall off the toilet" episode.

Put another way, I hurt my neck.

A few days later, my limbs became very weak, in the same way they had prior to my neck surgery. Kendra, my doctors, and I agreed that I shouldn't be left alone anymore. It would be too dangerous. I might fall again. Sometime in April, a night shift was added to my caregiving squad.

The first of the new recruits was Esperanza, a young Latina who filled my apartment with warmth, light, and humor. Right off, I told her to bring roller skates. She was skeptical, but ready to join in the fun. She brought her skates on her next shift and held on tight to the handles of my power chair as I pulled her around the neighborhood at dusk.

On a warm night in May, I awoke all at once and sat bolt upright. The clock said 2:30. I felt a powerful urge to watch TV. I turned it on. It was already tuned to one of 500 little-watched broadcast channels. And there it was, incontrovertible proof that Jung was right, that synchronicity is real. *The Elephant Man,* starring John Hurt, was just starting. Esperanza and I watched the movie until four.

It is the true story of John Merrick. I first read about him in the mid-seventies. It was just a blurb, really, but it gave me chills. I felt a strong kinship with him. At last, an account of someone who was truly disabled, someone who knew how it feels to try to run laps backwards as your classmates watch. When I read the biography a few years later, John Merrick became my blood brother. The book made me feel that I was not alone.

We watched as Anne Bancroft, playing an elegant Victorian actress, said to the hero, "Why, you are not a monster, Mr. Merrick. You are Romeo." She was talking directly to me.

At the end, Esperanza and I were sobbing.

∾

As I was getting out of bed one morning in June, a sudden jolt of electricity shot down my spine. The pain took my breath away. I lay back down and relaxed. It went away. I told myself to be calm, that it wouldn't happen again. Breathe deeply. Nothing to worry about. These things sometimes happen. A fluke. After a bit, after my heart had slowed, I tried to get up again.

Zot!

From my neck, right down my backbone. Like being electrocuted. A minute or so later, I tried a few tentative experiments and found that if I just relaxed, and didn't try to move at all, everything was okay, but as soon as I tensed up my neck, or tried to move, it went wild, crackling down my spine.

As I've said, complaining about pain rarely does any good. Besides, stoicism props up my sense of dignity. And I don't really like asking people for help, either. But just as there are limits to the power of the human will, so are there limits to stoicism, and to self-reliance. And I seemed to have reached those limits.

I called out for Patrick. He's the other half of my new 24-hour care team and now lives in the spare bedroom. He exemplifies the idea that intelligence is a tool that can be turned to any task. I'm lucky to have him as a friend and assistant. As soon as he came in the room, I asked him to call Kendra. She came right over and immediately called my neurologist, who recommended that we come in for a consultation that afternoon. I hesitated.

As I saw it, the professional surgical team's lifetime win-loss record on my home court, by which I mean on me, was about 3-5. Three wins, five losses. Past performance is no guarantee of future results, of course, but why would I bet on a team with such a lousy record? The odds just seemed too long.

So I said, "Wait. I. Might. Get. Better." After a bit of back and forth, Kendra reluctantly agreed to honor my wishes and wait.

It became my job to move as little as possible. Despite the pain, I didn't take any meds. I'd found that taking oxycodone is like inviting a vampire in as a houseguest. He readily accepts the invitation but can't take a hint when it's time to leave. He sticks around for supper.

The following day, my head became heavier and heavier, harder to lift. My shoulder and back muscles felt like they were going away. By the afternoon, my arms were becoming difficult to move, and my fingers clamped shut.

Then, early the next morning, two days after it had started, the feeling of electricity stopped. Suddenly. As though a switch had been thrown. And when that switch was thrown, an odd thing happened.

My body and my head were unplugged.

Not completely, but almost. My heart was still pounding, of course, and I was still breathing. But I couldn't sit up, hold my head up, or turn over, or even move my limbs. I could still move my hands a little, but I was numb from the neck down. It was as though a dentist had given me a huge shot of lidocaine in my neck. I could still try to say things, but not very successfully. Only a garbled, gurgling whisper came out.

As I lay there, looking at the ceiling, unable to move, I wasn't scared. Instead, I was wondering how the neurons and cells of my body had generated all that electricity. It had felt like the very force of life. And I was puzzled. Where had all that energy gone?

I knew that the stenosis had returned with a vengeance. My spinal cord was being squeezed hard by the same neck bones that had been fused and screwed together years before. The messages being sent from my brain to my muscles were being cut off at the pass in my neck. So, I couldn't move my limbs. Even the messages sent by that cluster of rogue nerve cells in my thalamus were being cut off. So, no more spasms. And the messages being sent from my body back to my brain were being ambushed, too. So, no more pain.

No spasms. No pain. A silver lining of sorts. Two silver linings, I guess you could say.

I seemed to have transitioned. Once a spastic, now, at the age of 65, I am a quadriplegic.

Does my life end like this?

I considered the implications. What if I can't write? What if I can't share my thoughts and feelings? What if I can't sing and dance? What would I do then? After all, I'm the one who said that you can dance anywhere, that anybody can dance, that everyone should dance. Would it be hypocritical of me to reconsider that position now? Given the circumstances?

And where is the hope?

It also occurred to me that while allowing surgeons to use DBS to try to cure me of dystonia, it had turned me into an unsuccessful traitor to the disability movement. Giving up now would surely make me a deserter.

For decades now, the question has always been, "What do I have to offer?" And there's always been an answer. Whether it was a play, a poem, a painting, or a performance, there was always something I could give. A counseling session, a seminar, or even a salamander. Always something.

What do I have to live for?

And I realized that there are still a few pressing items on my life's to-do list. Things that only I can do. For example, who else could tell this very story, if not me? The whole spastic transitioning into quadriplegic story? The panoramic view from here?

No one.

And even though I can't move, the force is still strong in me. I'm not going to give up. I'm not going to quit. Not here. Not now.

66

A Day at the Beach

Basking in the Sun, Not Moving a Muscle

Still Summer 2019

The foundation of the first tokamak fusion reactor is complete. So, in 2035, if everything goes exactly as planned, the world's first artificial sun will be ignited in the South of France.

The Peanut Butter Falcon **will open soon in a theater near you. Think of Huckleberry Finn reimagined as a young wrestler with Down syndrome.**

I'm stuck in bed. I have to live with it. That's the way it is.

I need a hospital bed. I get one placed in the middle of the living room. It has wheels and side rails and is endlessly adjustable, with a servomotor and all kinds of buttons. Instead of being isolated in the bedroom, I choose to be at the crossroads of the apartment, where everyone must pass, no matter where they're going. And my bed is perfectly positioned for a slumber party.

I need more help. As Patrick is already in the spare room, Wendy agrees to move into what was until recently my bedroom.

I soon learn that when your body does not feel and you cannot move it, the boundary between you and your surroundings blurs. In a way, you become your environment. So now I am not *in* the living room so much as I *am* the living room. Full time.

I am entirely in the hands of others. To move, I must be moved. People mishandle me, my rubbery form flopping this way and that. And I cannot help. I am dead weight. A sack of potatoes.

A hoyer lift, a sort of rolling crane fitted out with a cloth sling, is brought in so that I can be moved without anyone getting hurt. Hanging in its sling, I am like a dying fish scrunched up in a dip net. This isn't fun like a ride at Disneyland, or even like a golf cart or a power chair. Suspended here in this sling, bobbing, I feel like I'm a soloist in the Bolshoi's "special" sado-masochistic troupe.

It is *not* okay.

The Hoyer lift cuts me off from all human contact, which is what I need. A thigh to lie against, a torso to lean on, even a simple hug. This is what would help me. This is what I crave. Instead, here I am, being hoisted up in this rancid hammock.

"Does it feel okay, Neil?"

"Yeah," I say. I can't feel anything at all. I have no patience. Not anymore.

Eating is a chore. I try to drink lots of vitamin C. The skin on my face is flakey. And food collects around my mouth, especially in the corners, where red welts form. They sting. My face and eyes must be wiped constantly. There's more. I wet the bed. My groin is always damp. A rash appears, then spreads. It doesn't hurt, but it looks painful, angry. I must be gently cleansed several times each day.

This is not my idea of a good time.

When I was eight, I learned what it was to suddenly have a different body, a new body. I learned then that having a new body can change your outlook. Profoundly. It can change how you measure things. What was once a small thing can suddenly loom very large. Take freedom, for example. How do you measure freedom? To me, freedom now means being able to have a good bowel movement on a real toilet. If I am placed on the toilet just so, and I don't topple over, I am able to enjoy the kind of thrill that I imagine a lone climber feels when he stands on the summit of an icy peak, high in the Canadian Rockies, facing the wind, swaying slightly.

If I had three wishes, one of them would be that I could use a real toilet.

This is a bad dream; I can't wake up.

"Tell. Me. A. Story," I ask everyone.

I can't write. Progress on my book has slowed to a crawl. I'm not much help. I just can't do it.

~

Sometimes I have a poem in my mind that scratches on the inside of my mind, clambering to be let out. Now, more often than not, the scratching grows fainter and fainter, then stops.

Sometimes I reminisce. Across town is the old Unitarian Universalist Church. It has been a hangout for unkempt radicals since before I was born. During one summer in the early 80s, I'd go there for the singles' group on Friday nights. There was a girl named Rolann. Creamy skin and rosy cheeks. I used to help her buy the wine, cheese, and crackers for the meetings. A gallon of Gallo. I ended up being her boyfriend. She was Swedish, or maybe Norwegian. We would all play Password. Rolann and I were on the same team.

"Spirit."

"Ghost."

"Heart."

"Soul."

"Ding!"

When the meetings would break up around midnight, I would walk Rolann home through the empty streets. Then I'd head home. It was about a mile away. The streets were all mine. Roll, roll, roll. I was free. Zzzzzzzzzzz. Now it seems so dreamlike, so perfect. Idyllic.

～

I am reluctant to see a doctor. Friends and family hound me to go. A loving hounding, perhaps, but hounding, just the same.

I give in.

The specialist looks perplexed. My particular combination of paralysis, osteoarthritis, foraminal stenosis, and generalized dystonia must be new to him. He is half my age. He mumbles something about "wear and tear." It is clear that he has no idea what's going on with me. It is also clear that he thinks I know nothing. It does not occur to him to ask for my opinion. I'm neither surprised nor disappointed. I've concluded that no one knows what's going on with me, and that no one cares. He notices me watching him and averts his eyes. He sends me to be x-rayed.

The x-ray crew are overworked and baffled. I do not hand out George Clooney pictures. Those days are long gone. They transfer my inert form from the rolling bed to the x-ray table. Before lifting me, one of them counts.

"One … two … three!"

Some Eskimo villages celebrate the close of the whaling season by having a ring of people pull on the edges of a huge blanket, propelling the successful whaling captain up to 40 feet into the air. The people doing the pulling are called *nulluaqtit,* or "tossers." The event is usually called a blanket toss.

I am on the table. They try to bend my body in ways that my body does not bend. I try to tell them this, but they do not understand me. They are not really listening. They hurt my neck. They humiliate me. The x-rays are taken. Then the tossers transfer me back onto the rolling bed.

"One … two … three!"

I am back in the specialist's office. He studies the x-rays closely for several minutes, then turns to me.

"It would be an invasive surgery. We would go in from the front and insert a metal support into your neck. Due to the deterioration of both the bone and the covering of the spinal cord, the risk level is very high. Your paralysis could become irreversible. It is also possible that you wouldn't make it through the procedure. And, even if the surgery were successful, recovery would mean months in a rigid cervical collar, a lot of discomfort, and much pain. Medication would help, but on the other side of recovery, both the dystonia and osteoarthritis would be waiting."

As I listen, I think, "Give it to me straight, doc."

I must choose. Should I allow myself to once more be mutilated on the off chance that, after months alternating between unbearable pain and narcotic stupor, my spasms will reactivate and my joints will once again be free to constantly remind me of their inflamed and swollen state? Or should I continue to float on my back, gently drifting down life's stream, remembering, forgetting, a disembodied living room, numbly imagining, merrily dreaming? Not much of a choice.

In a slow whisper, I rasp, "No. More. Surgery. For. Me. Thanks. I'm. Good."

It's now about two months since the switch was thrown that disconnected my body from my head.

I wake up feeling uncomfortable and, without thinking about it, try to straighten my leg.

It moves!

67
It's Alive!

Regained Function

~

Late Summer 2019

The last VW Beetle has rolled off the assembly line in Puebla, Mexico.

Donald Trump expresses an interest in buying Greenland.

~

I CAN MOVE MY ARMS and legs again. Slowly, and without much force. No one seems to know why. Still, this gives me a feeling of hope. These days, whenever hope shows up at my door, I immediately fit him out in armor from head to toe, to prepare him for single combat with disappointment. Call it iron-clad hope.

A doctor prescribes some corticosteroid pills. They free up my limbs even more. And give me more energy.

Good. I've got work to do.

I must set up the living room. Everything must be very close, every movement as efficient as possible. Every second counts. Put the TV right there. And the computer right here, right next to me. Bluetooth will help. All fiber optic. Put the rolling writing desk right next to me. I must be able to reach everything easily. It must be uncluttered, with all the wires neatly bundled. Nothing in the way. No distraction. Ready for action.

This restored mobility means more time and energy for the book. Now we can make some real progress.

$\sim$

Writing the book has been a complicated process. Some of it is what I wrote long ago, word for word. Look for the spare lines that bend the rules. More often, while the passage may be based on what I wrote, it flows a bit more smoothly than my original draft. Be assured though, the thought that lies at the heart of even the wordiest paragraph is mine.

In late 2019, I began to write directly into the document, while my friend spent more time on the chat bar, making suggestions and observations. My sister Kendra and my brother Russell were valuable critics as well. Don't get the wrong idea, though: the choices that went into the final draft were mine. As a result, while I will be able to take credit for the book, I'll have to accept the blame as well. I've changed a few names when discretion seemed to call for it, but the rest is the way I remember it.

I must finish what I started.

$\sim$

My brother Roger, who lives and works in Berlin now, came to visit in late August. My living room became our private film festival. He had brought along *The Millenium Trilogy*, the Swedish films that start with *The Girl with the Dragon Tattoo*.

Near the end of the third movie, Lisbeth, she of the tattoo, seems to be out of danger at last. But then she goes to an old warehouse where she encounters her wicked half-brother, who tries to strangle her. She frantically tries to get away from him, then, in an act of desperation, she ducks between his gigantic legs and nails his feet to the floor with a nail gun. Although he is incapable of feeling pain, he can't move.

"You are in big trouble now, you freak!" Lisbeth yells.

She promptly calls both the police and her half-brother's nemesis, an outlaw biker, then leaves the warehouse before either of them arrives.

There's that word: *freak.*

There was a time when I would have objected to the term being used at all. Its sordid history would have lit up in neon: "See the caged geek at the freak show! Ten cents!"

I would have bristled. Lisbeth, of course, used the word not to label a person who had a disability, but rather to label a person who had what might be called a morality issue, someone who was, not to put too fine a point on it, evil. I mean, her half-brother really was quite nasty. Not in any metaphysical sense, of course, but the garden variety of evil that takes pleasure in causing others pain.

But I wasn't interested in whether freak was a politically correct word or whether someone might innocently be watching only to have their feelings hurt when Lisbeth blurted it out. I didn't bristle. Not a single hair. In fact, I enjoyed hearing her call him a freak and I enjoyed watching her nail his feet to the floor. The use of freak as a term of oppression was the furthest thing from my mind. I enjoyed all of it.

My big sister didn't approve of her younger brothers watching this movie, so full of torture, and evil, and revenge. She was sure that watching all the violence would harm us, psychologically, even spiritually. Her concern seemed misguided, puritanical, even a little funny. She's wrong. Seeing this story of an innocent young girl who is tortured and then dines on revenge was good for me.

It's like this. Violence is done to me every day. It is done on me every day. That's right: on me. I live it. I am disrespected. Every day. It is a form of violence. To be thought of as a retard, a monster, a freak. It is a kind of torture.

And if a film is done just right, with a great script, a talented cast, and a skilled director, a well-told story about a wronged good guy seeking and getting sweet revenge against the evil bad guy makes me laugh out loud and soothes my soul. Let the knives come out, let the blood flow. Let them scream. Go ahead. I don't care. I want justice, and I crave vengeance, and where's the harm if I let Steven Seagal get it for me every now and then? While I watch from the privacy of my own living room? Laid out here on my very own hospital bed? With my brother just in from Berlin? Eating some goddamn popcorn?

Best party ever.

Let the games begin.

～

I got out of bed again.

For the first time in months, I went outside, in my power chair, out onto the streets of Berkeley. A clear day. A caregiver was walking right behind me. Hovering. All those years of striving for independence, self-reliance, self-sufficiency, gone. Just like that. Up in smoke. Nice breeze, though.

After Roger left, my nephew's son, Logan, Wendy's grandson, came to visit. We immediately clicked. Wendy, Logan, and I would go jogging down the sidewalks of the neighborhood, under the arched domes of rustling autumn leaves.

In November, Logan left.

In December, the steroids started to lose their magic.

At the end of January, I watched motionless from my bed as hope slipped out the door. Unplugged again, paralyzed from the neck down, I float gently into February, turning slowly in an eddy of the current of time.

68

THE WALLS FALL AWAY

In the Home Stretch

March 2020

The coronavirus is on the loose and replicating itself in people everywhere.
All over the world, people have closed themselves securely in
their own homes.

I DON'T TRUST DOCTORS now. When I'm in the waiting room, I feel like a dog at the vet's. I do my best to appear calm, but I feel like I'm going to pee all over the floor any second. I'm 66 years old and when the receptionist says, "The doctor will see you now," I want to scream. My faith in the power of medicine has worn thin.

The steroids aren't working now. I cannot move. My fingers are all tied in a knot. Which means I can't write. How can I live like this? My sense of hope and purpose has always been tied to my ability to work. When I can work, I am up, at times even ecstatic. When I can't work, I am down, at times severely depressed. Without purpose, without a hope to cling to, I fall into despair.

All the beautiful words of my revolutionary poetry, about how love is dance and dance is life? They have lost all meaning to me. It's garbage. I'm garbage. I want out. Yes, I'm tired of the fight. This is too much to bear.

Am I really this exceptional fantastic spastic? Was I ever? Or am I just a wimp? Did I just fool myself in my attempt to be normal or "human" with all that pop psychology? Was I just playing empty word and mind games with myself? Trying to fool myself and anybody else who would fall for it? What if my whole career as an artist has been nothing more than a futile, foolish attempt to disguise and deny a grim reality? To me, right now, the only thing that seems real is to acknowledge death.

Right now, suicide sounds pretty good. I think about using a gun, but no, that would be too hard. Then I think about jumping out this window.

I broach the subject with Kendra. Just bringing the subject up helps a lot. I hate all that hiding behind bravery, that stiff upper lip crap. It feels liberating to be able to talk to someone about this.

"This. Is. Too. Much. To. Face. Ken. I. Need. Your. Help. I. Need. You. To. Help. Me. Jump. Out. That. Window." I start crying. The horror is out. I said it. Of course, no one would help me do that. It's an unreasonable request. I know that, but this isn't exactly a reasonable situation either, is it? I mean, this isn't a 50s sitcom where Dad can sit down with the boys in the final scene and give them just the right pep talk to keep them on the straight and narrow, is it? This isn't Disney. This isn't Shangri-La. This is real.

"Yes," says Kendra, "I understand. I think your wish for your life to be over is very reasonable. You've had a very good life. Rich and full. And with all of this happening to you now, it's perfectly reasonable that you would want it to be over." Now there are tears running down her cheeks, too. Her voice is trembling. "But you're not going to jump. It's out of the question. This is only the eighth floor and you'd probably just end up hurting yourself. You'd just make things worse. Besides, it would be too messy."

To which I think, "Jeez, Ken, you could have at least tried to talk me out of the whole idea."

Then Kendra tells me that in California it is legal for physicians to help people die neatly. It is called the "end of life option." She explains the steps involved and then tells me about another option: hospice.

Kendra invites some hospice people to my home. One of them is Dr. Sethi, whose countenance immediately reminds me of the Buddha. Right away, she senses that I am fed up with bureaucracy, and she keeps the talk between the two of us.

She tells me about joining hospice. Medicine could be prescribed that would make me as comfortable as possible. They could prescribe steroids and other meds in doses that, due to their potential long-term harmful side effects, aren't used in curative treatment. Counseling would be available to help me work through the issues that might arise. She also tells me about the regular nurses' and counselors' visits and about additional home assistance, for things like bathing. She is like a waiter at an upscale restaurant reciting today's luncheon specials. All upbeat, matter of fact, and maybe a little over-rehearsed. But when you sign up for hospice, she emphasizes, curative medicines and procedures stop.

To enroll in hospice, to say "yes" to Dr. Sethi's first offer, seems to me like giving in, like surrendering the little that remains of my independence. I fight the idea. I wrestle with it. Then it occurs to me that I would still get to decide what to order from the hospice menu, and when. I could also decide to quit hospice if I changed my mind. I'd still be in charge. In the end, even though it isn't really my style, I give in.

I join hospice.

So now the purpose of my medical care will no longer be to cure me or to prolong my life for as long as possible. No more neck or brain surgeries, and no iron lung for me. No heroic or artificial measures. And no cryogenic cylinder, either. Henceforth, the purpose of my medical care shall be much simpler. It will be to make me comfortable as I wait for natural death or, if I so choose, to exercise the "end of life option."

A few days later, a young neurologist tells me about the serious potential side effects of the prolonged use of high doses of steroids. She explains that the little pile of pills in front of me is a dose of corticosteroids twice as strong as the one I was last given, the dose that was so manifestly not up to the job. The look in her eyes and the tone of her voice suggest that she is concerned that these pills, taken together, may constitute an excessive, even dangerous, dose. Tellingly, she employs the word "frankly" twice.

"Do you still want to take this medicine?"

I fix my gaze on the young neurologist and raise one eyebrow. I take a second to study her unlined face, apparently untroubled by questions about meaning and nagging doubts about purpose. I then answer in my most forceful, gurgly whisper.

"Let's. Do. This."

I open my mouth very wide.

Later, one of my caregivers arrives. She is from Poland and has become a close friend. I tell her about my doubt and pain and about the medicine that could end my life. In her simple English she says, tenderly, "Don't think of that, Neil. Your soul is beautiful, deserved of great honor. Don't believe nothing else. Only this."

My heart opens. She is right. She continues. "So many people love you. It's because of who you are. They see. They feel your goodness. Your life is demonstration."

"Yes," I say. I sob silently. Would suicide be a form of betrayal? What am I supposed to do?

❧

Within a few days, the swelling around my spinal cord goes way down. The medicine is working.

Now I can move my arms and legs much better. Marching orders. The messages from my brain are getting through to my muscles. Let's dance. And, of course, random spasm commands and pain signals from a dozen joints are now flying freely up and down my spine as well.

My spirit soars. Boosted by an overdose of steroids.

I can move again. I can work again.

The streets outside my window are silent and empty. Quarantine. It's like a perfect dream.

I am in exactly the right place at precisely the right time. I have everything I need, cloistered here in my peaceful home. My roommate, Patrick, can find anything, fix anything, and figure out whatever needs to be figured out. Patrick solves problems. He has an encyclopedic memory and every tool we might ever need. He is Lewis to my Clark. I am on the home stretch. We're blazing a trail to the Pacific.

And miraculously, I can communicate, really communicate, at last. Patrick gets me a new, very powerful, very fast computer. It took 50 years for technology to do it, but I can now communicate reasonably well at a distance. I am connected to everyone from my past through Zoom. For the first time, I can meet with groups of people virtually. People who are all over the world, all talking with one another, together here on my computer screen. I feel free again.

I sleep well. No worries. I'm being fed good meals as I think, type, and reach out to my friends. Time does not hinder me now. My clock is ticking very slowly. My whole world is opening. I'm six years old again.

During the time that I was becalmed, observing and contemplating from my bed, my mind was busy below deck, quietly gathering and folding together all the corners of my life, arranging and joining the pieces of this fabric, layer upon layer. The doldrums are behind me now, and this newly sewn cloth is being unfurled. The mainsail is being raised, filling with wind. It is a shining tapestry.

My mind is clear.

I know it sounds odd, but I now know what is real. I know what is valuable. There are moments when I feel that these thoughts are not just mine. I feel that the universe is speaking through me.

69
No Net

The virus has run amok.
People have gone mad.
Hiding, hoarding, masking, marching.
Shouting, shooting, burning, looting.
Becoming reacquainted with death.
Things have come unglued.

~

I'm out of hospice. Three months ago, when I was first enrolled, it wasn't clear that I was going to die any time soon. And since hospice is supposed to be reserved for those with very little rope left, I had to ask myself once more, "Why me?"

They may have made an exception because I looked like I was ringing death's doorbell. I suppose I still do. After all, I have been functioning at full dystonic flex day after day for almost six decades now. Year after year. Procedure after procedure. All at full tilt. That's a lot of hard miles on a human body. Now, at 66 years old, I just look *so* different. And I suppose the fact that I was paralyzed at the time of the interview made my portrayal of a weary pioneer about to cross the Great Divide all the more convincing.

I didn't die, of course. In fact, I kept feeling better. Feeling happier. Writing more. Doing more art. I'm not losing weight. I'm not stuck in bed. I'm out, and about. I'm very active. Cruising the streets daily. Streets made empty by the news of Covid 19 that is scaring the whole world. But I'm not afraid. I feel at peace. And very much alive.

Then, as weeks turned into months, I began to detect impatience. It was as though the hospice people were tapping their feet in unison and saying, "If you're not dying, Mr. Marcus, why are you enrolled in hospice? Mmmm?" *Tap, tap tap.* "Mmmm?"

I began to feel some small measure of guilt being enrolled in hospice. After all, one mustn't hog all the health care resources. Just wouldn't be right. There are people who need them more. Of course, no one would dare be so straightforward with me as to suggest that I revoke my enrollment, but Kendra and I talk it over and we agree that, yes, I should ask to be discharged. And, as they discharge me, once more they call me "Sweetie."

I'm good, thanks. I'm living well. They offer me care that makes me as comfortable as possible. Just normal meds, normal doses. I'll try that. I now know that my expectations of hospice had been too high. And I don't need to seek out death. It will find me soon enough, anyway. Besides, my book isn't done. I have to finish my book. It's a blueprint. A roadmap.

～

July 15, 2020

I watched an old video from the 80s. I was dancing in a big ballroom. In my prime. It shocked me to see myself like that. It was a talent show and I was acting like Travolta strutting his stuff. Only my stuff was stuff nobody had seen before or would even think of as being stuff.

I knew what I was doing, though. Or thought I did. With every gesture, every jerk, every stretch, and every fall, I was saying, "Yes, I'm spastic. I cannot not be spastic. And know this: There is beauty in this spasticity, beauty that has been deliberately overlooked. And if I did not get up here and show this beauty to you, it might never be seen. It would be as though it did not exist."

But as I watched, I was seeing myself much more as others had seen me then. I think the distance of time and experience and the changes in me have given me the ability to better understand what was going on in the minds of that audience as they watched me dance. And I think they saw one of young men in Africa who crawl down unpaved village streets on withered legs. And I think they were watching the carnival geek rattle the bars of his cage as he howled. I now think that as they watched me dance my spastic dance, many of them were saying to themselves,

"I don't know if this is art, but that is one crazy son of a bitch."

❧

April 2021

For months now, my body has been AWOL. If my motor skills were once problematic, now they're more or less non-existent. For example, when I tell my arm to rise, usually only the elbow makes it off the bed. Sometimes I can pinch a napkin between my thumb and the knuckle of my forefinger. Sometimes I can't. And I can't sit up. A belt holds my torso upright, but it has to be adjusted several times each day as my body tends to slide out of my chair. I can still talk, but not clearly, judging by the number of "sorry, I didn't quite catch that" responses.

When most people grow impatient, they fidget. When sleep proves elusive, they toss and turn. Not me. I can do neither. Like Mark O'Brien, I have been dragooned by a biological press gang and sent to sea, floating flat on my back, meditating by default, an involuntary yogi. I have had a lot of time to drift and think.

As a spastic, I viewed the human pageant from a seat way off to one side of the theater. From that angle, I saw things that others simply couldn't. As a paralyzed person, I now see that same show as though from a great distance, like a live video feed looking back from a spaceship as it escapes the gravity of the earth. From here, things look very different.

Borders are imaginary lines that arbitrarily divide people in countless ways. From this distance, all such lines cease to exist. Similarly, ideas that seem to be in conflict can be seen as two sides of the same small coin. Opposing ideas share a common border. Contradictions vanish.

And there is no such thing as illness. It is a categorical illusion.

~

July 2021

Now that the subject has been broached, I feel compelled to tell you about my experiences with time portals.

I've had these experiences in several different settings, but they have occurred most often on my visits to the swimming pools and aquariums that have those dimly lit tunneled walkways that curve gently down to giant windows that look out into bright, clear water.

For example, this is Solano College. I swim in this pool several days a week after work. On my own. In private. Free and easy. It is my joy.

And this? This is the aquarium in Seattle. It has a similar feel to the school's pool, despite the sea life. Notice the soothing indirect lighting and the way even the smallest sound has its own echoes. That is a giant octopus.

When I visit these places, I often get confused. Not always, but often. I have to ask myself: where am I? Is this an aquarium? Or am I somewhere else entirely? And what time is it? What year? I can't tell. Not the where, not the when.

I think this is time travel. Maybe.

This has been happening to me more and more lately. And I don't think this is an aquarium.

⌇

Summer, 2021

When I first got back from Silver Pines Camp, I thought, "Why is this happening to me?"

I wracked my brain. Bizarre explanations suggested themselves, most of them drawn from comic books or science fiction. Have aliens taken over my mind? Am I possessed by an ancient demon? Are there little bugs eating my brain? Is the disembodied spirit of a long-dead witch doctor toying with me? All these explanations seemed more likely than the psychologist's idea that I needed to be toughened up, but none of them rang true, either. In the mind of an eight-year-old, rational explanations for an unusual event are often made to stand in line with all the other possible explanations to wait their turn.

Late one evening, I was watching TV alone. The house was dark and my parents were asleep. They strictly monitored my viewing, so I had to turn the volume way down and sit real close to the screen. They watched boring stuff like the evening news. In my world, ghosts were at the top of the news and monsters were the celebrities. In my world, when you got scared, it wasn't because you had an overactive imagination, it was because something very real was happening that was truly frightening. In my world, everything was not all rosy.

The show that night was *Horror Night Saturday Special.* To me, watching it felt more like research than entertainment. To me, the horror movies it showed were more like documentaries. The monsters on these shows, I know now, can be seen as the misunderstood, marginalized, and alienated of society. I know now that it is not these monsters who are evil, but those who torment them. At eight, I didn't know that, but I felt that hidden in these movies was a key that I had to find. A key that I needed.

On that particular night, a grainy, black-and-white movie was on. One of the characters was an old gypsy fortune-teller. The actress playing the part was Maria Ouspenskaya. She had been my mom's drama teacher. Her picture is in my mom's college scrapbook. That she was in the film made me feel that something far deeper was going on here than mere coincidence. I got goosebumps. Forces were at work. I felt sure that this old movie was being broadcast at this exact time to provide an answer to the gnawing question: why me?

The movie was *The Wolf Man.*

As it ended, I watched the credits, then the flag waving as the national anthem played. My eyelids were heavy, but I felt very much awake. The channel went off the air. The screen filled with electronic snow, but I didn't turn the TV off. I didn't look away. I stared as thoughts coalesced.

Before I saw *The Wolf Man,* all of the explanations I'd considered for what I would later learn to call dystonia defined it as an affliction. Whether the cause was physiological, psychological, spiritual, I was the afflicted. The helpless victim. It was a given.

The Wolf Man possessed a power that was missing from my reality. I could feel it. I felt comforted by it and drawn to it. I found myself attracted to the Wolf Man's menace. I identified with him. The crucial scene was where the old gypsy psychic consoled the Wolf Man and told him of his destiny. That scene suggested a new explanation for what was happening to me.

What if I am not a victim, but a hero, who is being offered the honor of undertaking a holy quest? What if this is not an affliction, but an ancient mantle passed down through the ages that, at a great but bearable cost, conveys deep knowledge and awesome power to the one who chooses to wear it? What if I am being called upon to be a Champion of the Light who must fight to save Humankind from Darkness? What if I am being called upon to be a savior?

While I no longer wonder if I am the messiah and dystonia is the cross upon which I am nailed, I know that the Wolf Man's story helped shape me as I grew up. I carried it with me. To this day, it is part of the personal mythology that sustains me.

There is a power in disability that most people are not aware of. Those who are aware of this power almost never speak of it.

Here is what I learned from the Wolf Man.

Disability isn't all bad.

∼

Fall 2021

Sitting in my chair, looking out the window, watching the sun set over the Bay, I'm alone, for the moment at least. I glance down at the penny my dad put on the tracks almost sixty years ago. I touch it and sigh, then smile.

I'm not touching this flattened penny for luck. I've had more luck than most people. I touch it now as a gesture of gratitude to everyone who helped me, who showed me the way. I touch it as a reminder that there are still millions of people, young and old, who are trying to hide and looking for someone to show them the way out. Touching it helps me to keep these people in mind, and everything in perspective. Culture, at its best, supports people, and lifts them up. Art, in my view, does the lifting. I hope I've done my part.

Afterwords

What would you do if you were a healthy, happy child and, out of the blue, you lose control of your body? Your muscles are gripped by persistent, random spasms. You graduate to a wheelchair. People struggle to understand you when you speak. Even swallowing food is hard. Your body often curls into a tight ball.

What would you do?

Picture two boys.

The first boy wakes up on his bed one morning to discover that during the night he has been transformed into a spastic. Not just a slightly errant right hand, mind you, but every muscle in open rebellion. Full throttle dystonia.

What does he do? Well, he hides it. Which can only mean he hides himself. He hides because when others see him, he can see the fear in their faces, and he can see their revulsion and their pity. He hides because he feels fear, too, and then shame. So he hides in his room, watching television, passively observing the electronic images of people living out there in the world. He discovers that as long as he stays there the shame and fear are under his control, not gone, but tamped down. He can stand it. He is safely shut in.

The boy grows older, living at home, sheltered from the outer world, safe from fear and shame. He does not give love and is not open to receiving love except within his narrow world. He has no accomplishments, no adventures, no triumphs. And so, as the years pass, he continues, living with his aging parents, then, later, in an assisted living facility, all alone now, and sadder.

Years later, living in a nursing home, he is a castaway. And when he passes, as we all must, he passes unnoticed, in silence. Not even a ripple in the pond. As though he had never been here at all.

About that other boy.

He also wakes up one morning to find that he has become a spastic. Head to foot. Initially, he feels the same fear and shame as the first boy.

But, he decides to face his fear and stare down his shame. He looks them both right in the eye. He then wills himself out into the world. He seeks out people. And he helps the people he meets overcome the fear, pity, and revulsion that they feel.

And if he had done only that, and nothing more, it would have been a lot.

But then he makes up his mind that he will love people. Not just some people, but everyone. Even people who think that they do not deserve love, even those who say they don't want it. And he decides to seek out love and to accept it when it is offered, and to accept all the risks and pains that accompany giving and receiving love.

He makes up his mind to seek out adventure. He wants to experience all that this beautiful and dangerous world has to offer, tackling every opportunity and challenge that his dystonic body can handle. He jumps right in. Off the high dive. Down the rapids. A real daredevil.

And if that were the end of it, it would be remarkable.

But.

Now he chooses to take on the world itself. This world that makes life so difficult for so many people must be changed, he decides. This world should become a place free from fear, pity, shame, and revulsion.

And so, he works at it. Day after day. Year after year. It is like he is building the Great Pyramid. Stone by stone. For fifty years. To get the message out. Showing that disability can be an enriching and positive part of everyday life. Showing that there is nothing to fear.

He writes. Spreading his message. Letter by letter. Page by page. Newsletters, articles, books of poems, plays, an autobiography.

He creates drawings, paintings, and cartoons. All with lines, shapes, and ideas that surprise.

He acts. In and out of his chair. Falling sometimes, and always rising. On stage, on television, on the big screen. Dystonic energy on full display.

He dances and poses for photographers and painters, showing all the world that disability is part of the beauty of the world. A new genre, a new aesthetic, a new art. A new world.

Behold!

He takes the stage. Then bigger and bigger stages. In front of hundreds, thousands, and finally, millions of people. To make the world better, more caring, more inclusive, more loving. Helping humanity take its next step up. Above pity. Above shame. Above fear. Helping us to evolve. Showing the way.

That he does this at all is amazing. But what is truly amazing is that he does it with such charismatic spastic style. He makes friends. Thousands of them. At countless casual dinner parties, he captivates the table with necessarily pithy observations that light up the conversation and ignite laughter. People at neighboring tables often glance sidelong in wonder at this slightly grungy bon vivant with his jagged frame and flashing eyes, asking themselves, "Who is this guy?"

He lives life to the fullest.

With warmth and a sharp wit.

With a good-natured stubbornness.

With a mischievous, open-hearted generosity.

With spastic grace and boundless optimism.

With genius.

And, most importantly,

With love.

Ladies and gentlemen … Neil Marcus.

∼

In mid-November of 2021, Neil endured two bouts of high fever accompanied by continuous and severe muscle spasms. Each lasted more than ten hours. The second bout burned even hotter than the first. No one knows why.

On November 17, 2021, at 11:04 AM, Neil passed away. Kendra was there with him, as was his visiting nurse. Patrick was in the other room. About a half hour later, three small earthquakes shook the building. Right on cue.

—S. H. Chambers

NEIL MARCUS
(1954-2021)

1954
Neil Marcus, the youngest of five children, born in White Plains, NY

1961
Marcus family moves to Ojai, CA

1962
Dystonia symptoms appear; Neil attends sleepover summer camp

1963
Diagnosed with *dystonia musculorum deformans*

1967
Remission from dystonia

1968
Begins boarding at Ojai Valley School tenth grade; dystonia remission ends and depression follows

1969
Learns about co-counselling

1971
Graduates high school, class valedictorian; attends Fairhaven College, (Western Washington University) in Bellingham, WA

1974
Attends Moorpark College; writes column and feature stories for *Ojai Valley News*

1976
Works as Enabling Aid counselling disabled students at Solano Community College; writes and edits newsletter, *Rising Tide*, for disabled community; establishes peer counseling program and leads counseling workshops

1979

Moves to Berkeley, CA; receives crash course in identity politics; enrolls in computer programming class at Center for Independent Living

1970-90's

Writes *Complete Elegance*, a counseling journal, and *Special Effects*, a zine featuring writing and artwork (graphics, punk-rock typography, and concrete poetry), mixing stories from Berkeley's Independent Living movement with philosophical reflections and notes to Buckminster Fuller; writes *Fantastic Spastic* zine

1980

Quits computer programming

1985

Roger creates dramatic audio recording of Neil's diary entries

1987

Self-publishes *The Princess and The Dragon*, a disabled fable; Roger shares their recording with producer/director Rod Lathim of Access Theater, resulting in the production of *Storm Reading*

1988

Storm Reading debuts at Lobero Theatre in Santa Barbara. Neil and Roger TV interview with Maria Shriver, on *Sunday Today*

1988-96

Storm Reading goes on tour; Neil performs the show more than 300 times

1989

Excerpts of *Storm Reading* with Neil and Roger filmed for the Kennedy Center's *From the Heart: The First International Very Special Arts Festival*, which is aired on national television

1990

Stars in *Speaking Through Walls*, award-winning documentary directed by Anthony Edwards and co-produced with Shawn Hardin about Access Theatre and *Storm Reading* tour

1992

Neil and *Storm Reading* win *Drama-Logue Magazine*'s Best Leading Actor and Best Ensemble Awards

1993

Storm Reading voted one of Los Angeles' top 10 plays of the year; Neil receives Medal of Honor from UN Society of Writers for outstanding achievement in play writing

1996

Live audience filming of *Storm Reading*

1998

Neil appears on episode of television show *ER*

2000's

Guest lecturer at University of California, Berkeley, and co-teacher of "Disability and Digital Storytelling" with Professor Sue Schweik

2004

Interviewed by Regional Oral History Office at University of California, Berkeley for a project about artists with disabilities

2006

Invited by painter Riva Lehrer of Chicago Art Institute to display paintings in "Disability in Contemporary Art" show at Chicago Cultural Center

2008

Cripple Poetics by Petra Kuppers and Neil Marcus (Homofactus Press), a book of the authors' romantic correspondence

2009

Publishes essay in *Research in Drama Education: The Journal of Applied Theatre and Performance*; works with University of Michigan professor Petra Kuppers on the Olimpias Performance Research Project, an artist collective spotlighting performers with disabilities

2014

Smithsonian National Museum of American History commissions Neil to write poem and create video for online exhibition, "EveryBody: An Artifact History of Disability in America"

2018

30th anniversary performance of *Storm Reading* at Lobero Theatre

2019

Loses mobility, confined to bed

2020

Accepts hospice care

2021

Neil dies at his home in Berkeley

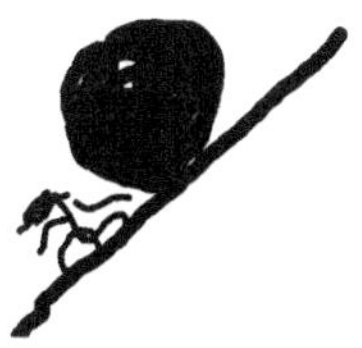

Learn More About Neil

~

Storm Reading photos, videos, audio, and press clippings on Access Theatre:
https://atarchives.wordpress.com/storm-reading/

Los Angeles Times article about *Storm Reading:*
https://www.latimes.com/archives/la-xpm-1989-03-30-ve-736-story.html

It just takes one: TV interview with Maria Shriver:
https://www.youtube.com/watch?v=GATf_nuFTgU

University of California Berkeley's Regional Oral History Office interviews of Neil Marcus:
https://digitalassets.lib.berkeley.edu/roho/ucb/text/marcus_neil.pdf

Smithsonian Institute's "EveryBody: An Artifact History of Disability in America":
- **https://americanhistory.si.edu/explore/stories/bodyfree-domart-rethinking-disability-through-art**
- **https://everybody.si.edu/place**
- **https://www.si.edu/object/neil-marcus-disabled-country%3Ayt_e8CLrv8dd-E**

Online Archive of California Collection – Neil Marcus papers:
https://oac.cdlib.org/findaid/ark:/13030/c81g0s05/admin/

Scholar.google.com – search for "Neil Marcus disability"

New York Times obituary:

https://www.nytimes.com/2021/12/28/arts/neil-marcus-dead.html

Accessibility.com obituary:

https://www.accessibility.com/blog/all-eyes-on-neil-marcus-a-champion-of-disability-visibility-through-artistry

Tribute to Neil Marcus on Disability Visibility Project's website:

https://disabilityvisibilityproject.com/2022/01/09/reading-storms-embracing-life-a-remembrance-of-neil-marcus/

KPFA 94.1 Memorial for Neil Marcus:

https://kpfa.org/episode/pushing-limits-june-3-2022/

Acknowledgments

~

I am grateful to all those who have contributed to the publication of Neil's autobiography. A few people deserve special mention because of their outsized contribution to the final book.

I want to extend my special thanks to S. H. Chambers, who spent years working with Neil and his archives to put together this inspiring book, and two more years with me providing guidance as I navigated the editorial process. Your good nature and great sense of humor went a long way to sustain Neil and motivate this project.

Thank you, brother Roger Marcus, for your thoughtful suggestions and for your memories of working with Neil. I also appreciated your photos capturing Neil in his Fred Astaire moments.

Thank you, brother Russell Marcus, for your good suggestions throughout.

For the finer details of publication, I am indebted to Minju Chang who took the lead as we moved from manuscript to print. Your unparalleled research skills and eagle-eyed attention to detail were invaluable.

I owe my deep gratitude to Renata Galindo, talented illustrator and designer, for keeping me on track, for your infinite patience and dedication to the project. Thank you for your brilliant ideas and enthusiasm.

And thank you to Liz Lank for the close attention you paid to the printed words and for keeping the book consistent.

Many thanks to Tracy Maurer for sharing her marketing skills and guiding me in my attempts to spread the word to readers far and wide.

And thank you, Rod Lathim, for being a staunch defender and ally of Neil and contributing photos, comments, and connections to help us spread the word.

Thank you, Devva Kasnitz, for your thoughtful feedback and for your enthusiastic help in connecting Neil's book to educators and beyond.

I also acknowledge the talented photographers who managed to capture Neil's generous spirit in the photos we used to show off Neil's talents. Thank you, Gary Ivanek, Mel Hofmann, Brenda Prager, and Petra Kuppers, for allowing us to use your fine photos showing Neil in all his aspects.

Special thanks to Anthony Edwards, Rod Lathim, and Devva Kasnitz for their kind and thoughtful words about Neil and for allowing us to print them here.

So many friends and family have offered thoughtful comments, giving me confidence to move forward with publishing Neil's book. To acknowledge everyone individually would fill another book. Please know that I appreciate and thank you all for your time and support throughout.

Below is a short list of people who generously shared reactions and suggestions as I made my way forward. Without you I could not have completed the task.

Adam Cotton

Agnieszka Nowick

Andrea Bersamin

Anthony Edwards

Catherine Signorelli

Chip Romer

David Seltzer

Deborah Massell

Dystonia Medical Research Foundation

Jerrie Lore

Karyn Fischer

Leslie Martin

Melina Bersamin

Paul Lore

Patrick Goodspeed

Sandy Gleysteen

Sidsel Millerstrom

Sylvia Perera

Wendy Marcus

—Kendra Marcus

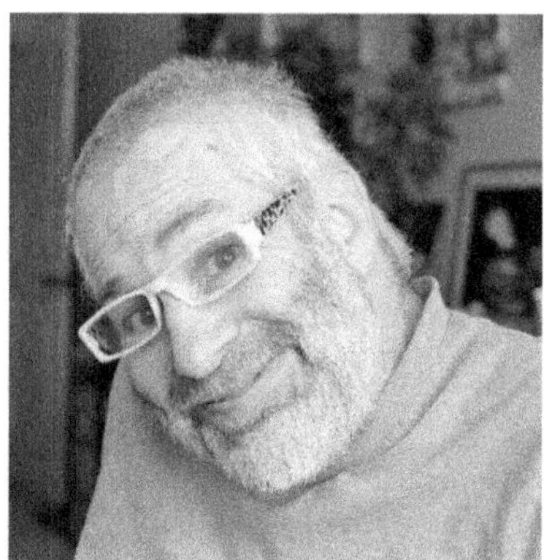

photo courtesy Mel Hofmann

Neil Marcus described himself as "a poet, humorist, writer, actor, and adventurer—a fantastic spastic creatively endowed with disability." He is best known for his groundbreaking autobiographical play, *Storm Reading*, which he performed across the nation from the Kennedy Center in Washington DC to the Doolittle theater in Los Angeles. He was commissioned to write a poem on disability by the Smithsonian Institute. He has been interviewed by Maria Shriver on *Sunday Today*, Linda Wertheimer on NPR's *All Things Considered*, and multiple hosts on KPFA radio. He leaves the world a legacy of creativity, political action and community building.

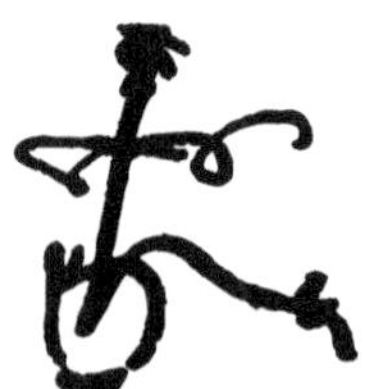

This image, painted by Neil, represents the
artistry, vitality, and beauty of the disabled life.